# Minimizing Medical Mistakes:

*The Art of Medical Decision Making*

# Minimizing Medical Mistakes:

*The Art of
Medical Decision Making*

## Richard K. Riegelman, M.D., Ph.D.

Professor of Health Care Sciences and Medicine, George
Washington University School of Medicine and Health
Sciences; Attending Physician, George Washington
University Hospital, Washington, D.C.

**Little, Brown and Company**
**Boston/Toronto/London**

Library of Congress Catalog Card No. 90-62669

ISBN 0-316-74523-5

Printed in the United States of America
SEM

# *Contents*

# *Preface*

*"The essence of learning is not merely doing but thinking about what one is doing."*

Gale and Masden [1], 1983

Medical decision making is easy! All clinicians have to do is get the facts right, order the appropriate tests, make the correct diagnosis, know the treatment of choice, and see that it's done! If only it were so simple, clinicians could readily be replaced by computers and robots. Every practicing clinician knows, and most medical students soon learn, that it is not that simple when put into practice.

As we shall see, despite our best efforts lots of things can and do go wrong in medical practice. Most clinicians, patients, and even lawyers acknowledge that everyone makes mistakes. Acknowledging our own mistakes, however, does not come easily. We may fear that our bad outcomes will be called mistakes and our mistakes will be called negligence. In an effort to make this process easier and less painful, *Minimizing*

*Medical Mistakes: The Art of Medical Decision Making* develops a framework for analyzing the reasons for undesirable results and provides suggestions for preventing their occurrence.

In *Minimizing Medical Mistakes* we refer to all less-than-desired outcomes as undesirable results. We then divide undesirable results into bad outcomes and mistakes. Bad outcomes imply that, knowing what we know now, we would not have done things differently. When a mistake has occurred, the implication is that we should have done things differently. Bad outcomes do not imply responsibility on the part of the physician, while errors or mistakes do imply responsibility. Errors or mistakes, as opposed to bad outcomes, are preventable.

We distinguish two basic types of errors that occur in the practice of clinical medicine: errors of ignorance and errors of implementation. Errors of ignorance imply that the clinician did not have the necessary knowledge to draw the correct conclusion or carry out the correct treatment. In *Minimizing Medical Mistakes*, we treat errors of ignorance as due to problems getting up to speed, staying up to speed, and knowing your own speed limit. Despite the fears of medical students, errors of implementation rather than errors of ignorance are the most common errors that occur and are the focus of much of the book. Errors of implementation imply problems utilizing what we know and applying it to the tasks of diagnosis and therapy.

The basic aim of this book is to provide a framework for analyzing errors of implementation and distinguishing them from errors of ignorance and bad outcomes. Errors of implementation are analyzed using mnemonics made up of the first letter of each step in the diagnostic or SHADE process, the therapeutic or PESTER process, and the TRUST process of developing a doctor-patient relationship. As we identify what can go wrong suggestions are made for minimizing these occurrences.

*Minimizing Medical Mistakes* begins by looking at the errors of implementation that occur in the diagnostic or SHADE process. The steps of symptom, hunch, alternatives, disease, and explanation are examined to identify the rules of thumb or heuristics that we use to get the job done. We will also examine the problems or biases that are inherent in the application of these rules of thumb.

Next, we examine the therapeutic or PESTER process. We look at the types of errors that occur in each step in the therapeutic process; including problems with prediction, effectiveness, safety, therapeutic decisions, execution of therapy, and reflection upon the results.

Having looked at the basic steps in diagnosis and treatment and examined what can go wrong in each, we turn our attention to the doctor-patient relationship, which is analyzed by looking at the steps in obtaining TRUST through therapeutic relationships, uncertainty sharing, and truth. Again we attempt to understand what should occur and what can go wrong.

In the last chapter, a flowchart presents the steps for categorizing undesirable results. Finally, we pause at the end of the book to take a look at how we can deal with and accept our own errors and ultimately face our own fallibility.

The goal of medical education according to Sir William Osler is, "to give a man his direction, point him the way, and furnish him with a chart, fairly incomplete for the voyage ..." [2]. Over the years Osler's chart has been filled in with new roads, whole new towns, and many more ways to get lost. *Minimizing Medical Mistakes* aims to help you chart your way around and, if necessary, out of those blind alleys.

Ultimately, we cannot eliminate mistakes or errors, but we can learn to minimize their occurrence, contain their consequences, and learn from those that do occur. By facing our own fallibility, we will be able to practice the art of medical decision making.

**R.K.R.**

1. Gale J, Masden P. *Medical Diagnosis from Student to Clinician.* Oxford: Oxford University, 1983. P. 158.
2. Osler, Sir William. *Aphorisms* from *His Bedside Teachings and Writings.* In WB Bean, (Ed.). New York: Henry Schuman, 1950. P. 36.

# *Acknowledgments*

During the more than ten years that it took to complete *Minimizing Medical Mistakes*, a large number of people have stimulated my thinking, provided essential critiques, and sustained my desire to see this project through. I would especially like to thank several people who played pivotal roles in this prolonged process. Gail Povar's insights, ideas, and willingness to read and reread have been enormously helpful. Tom Moore's thoughtful input helped me make key decisions about how to structure and orient the book. Arthur Elstein's input into an early manuscript provided essential guidance. Jackie Glover's review of the chapters relating to decision making and fallibility contributed significantly to the book's approach. A number of the ideas and approaches Jim Blatt uses in teaching have been generously donated to the book. Eve Bargmann and Scott Schroth's reviews helped confirm the clinical relevance of the basic approach.

As always, my wife Linda's support not only sustained me through the ups and downs of writing, but her ideas provided new approaches when I ran into blind alleys. Large numbers of friends and relatives also read early versions and contributed important ideas.

The reactions of second, third, and fourth year medical students, as well as residents at the George Washington University Medical Center, have been key to developing this book. Sally Santen was especially helpful in reading and re-reading the book.

I would also like to thank Annette Williams-Bishop for her competent and persistent work in putting together the manuscript and Maureen Flaherty, who helped organize the project.

It is always a pleasure to work with the editorial and marketing staff at Little, Brown's Medical Division. Their encouragement and advice have made an important contribution to this book.

Last but not least are my patients. The opportunity to participate in their care over the last decade has given me the opportunity to understand their expectations, hear their concerns, and gain a perspective on what medical care can provide, as well as its limitations. I am grateful for their help and inspiration.

# Raising the SHADE on the Diagnostic Process

# 1

# *Introduction*

Let us begin by taking a look at George Williams, a new patient making his first visit to your office.

George Williams is a 30-year-old white male who came to the office because of a five-week history of episodes of pain in the "pit of his stomach." The pain tends to occur before meals and is relieved by eating. Mr. Williams now seeks care because he has begun to "wake up in the middle of the night with the same pain." He has not attempted any therapy. When asked directly, he acknowledges "on occasion" drinking five to six martinis on a weekday with "a little more" on weekends. He does not use aspirin, other over-the-counter medications, or caffeine containing drinks regularly. He does not smoke cigarettes and has not had severe stresses in his personal or professional life. The pain he is experiencing does not radiate to other locations, and it is not associated with nausea, vomiting, changes in his bowel movements or other symptoms. During the physical examination he has a negative test for occult blood in the stool. His physical examination is within normal limits except for mild tenderness with palpation over the area of abdominal pain.

This patient has a commonly occurring pattern of disease. When approaching this and many types of patient problems, clinicians have been shown to utilize a remarkably uniform approach. Let us take a look at the steps involved in this process. We will demonstrate how a clinician might apply this process to this patient with stomach pain. We will then examine what is required for effective use of this approach to diagnosis when confronted with the complexity of clinical practice. In presenting and remembering this approach to diagnosis, we will construct the mnemonic SHADE by using the first letters of key words that describe the steps in the diagnostic process.

The SHADE approach to diagnosis consists of five steps that serve to generate and test a clinician's hypothesis or hunch about the patient's diagnosis. These steps are:

**S**ymptom: Focus on a chief complaint
**H**unch: Generate an early or initial hypothesis
**A**lternatives: Develop a differential diagnosis or list of alternatives
**D**isease: Disease identification by testing the hypothesis
**E**xplanation: Assess underlying cause and relate the patient's symptom to the identified disease(s)

## STEP 1. SYMPTOMS: FOCUSING ON A CHIEF COMPLAINT

When a physician is confronted with a new patient anything could be wrong. The whole universe of problems and diseases is possible at the initiation of a patient encounter. To focus on and accurately define the nature of the patient's problem, clinicians traditionally seek to identify the most important symptom or problem that brings the patient to medical care. This is called the patient's "chief" or "presenting complaint." Ideally the formulation of a chief complaint narrows and focuses the patient's and physician's attention on the reason for the patient's visit and the goal of the encounter. Under ideal circumstances the clinician's attention is concentrated on exactly the situation that is most urgent to the patient. This principal symptom then serves as the focus or pivot for the subsequent diagnostic process.

Our patient's chief symptom is pain in the "pit of the stomach." He seeks care now because he has been "awakened in the middle of the night with the same pain." Thus, focusing on the stomach pain as the principal symptom allows the clinician to focus on a diagnostically useful symptom that is central to the patient's concerns and to the patient's purpose for seeking care.

## STEP 2. HUNCHES: EARLY HYPOTHESIS GENERATION

In the process of obtaining data concerning the patient's chief complaint, clinicians almost routinely, and often subconsciously, formulate tentative ideas or hunches about what is wrong. Clinicians often instantly and intuitively match the patient's symptoms with the pattern of disease stored in the clinician's memory. Hunches are such a natural part of clinical thinking that many clinicians have great difficulty avoiding jumping to conclusions. It's not easy or desirable to suppress one's hunches, but it is important to distinguish a hunch from a conclusion. A hunch or hypothesis plays an important role by allowing the whole of medical training and experience to be brought to bear on a patient's problem from the beginning of the encounter. The process of hypothesis generation allows physicians to convert the open-ended question "what could be producing the chief complaint" to a more easily approached question "does the patient have disease X."

In the case of our patient with stomach pain, the location and timing of the pain makes most students and physicians immediately think of duodenal ulcer. The pain of duodenal ulcers is usually well localized to the epigastric region, the midportion of the upper abdomen. Duodenal ulcer pain usually occurs when the ulcer is exposed to stomach acid before meals and in the middle of the night. Food characteristically relieves the pain by temporarily stopping the irritating effects of unopposed stomach acid. Thus, this patient's problem fits well with the classic pattern of duodenal ulcer. The clinician is now faced with the manageable question "does the patient have a duodenal ulcer"?

## STEP 3. ALTERNATIVES: DEVELOPING A DIFFERENTIAL DIAGNOSIS

Repeated experience and formal training have taught most physicians to be skeptical of their initial hypothesis and seek further data to confirm or refute their initial hunches. This list of alternatives, or differential diagnosis, plays an important role by forcing the clinician to focus on other possible diseases. The differential diagnosis helps structure the questions that must still be answered in order to accept or reject the initial hunch or hypothesis.

Clinicians, like most other human beings, can usually contend with no more than five alternatives simultaneously. Clinicians, therefore, must use a great deal of judgment in selecting from an extensive list of possible diseases those conditions that should be under active consideration. The formulation of a limited number of active alternatives helps clinicians rapidly extract and apply their knowledge and experience to the patient's problem. It thus helps structure the task of collecting further data designed to rule in or rule out the presence of a particular disease.

In Mr. Williams' case there is a strong likelihood of duodenal ulcer. The high prevalence of duodenal ulcers, plus the pattern of his symptoms compatible with duodenal ulcer, support this hypothesis. Despite the evidence suggesting a duodenal ulcer, however, physicians usually recognize that other possibilities exist. Gastritis is another distinct possibility. Less likely, but still possible, is pancreatitis. A benign or even cancerous gastric ulcer is also a possibility since the pattern of pain in gastric ulcers can mimic duodenal ulcer. Other less likely possibilities are gallstones and pancreatic cancer.

Faced with a long list of possibilities, physicians must initially consider only a limited number of active possibilities. For instance, in this 30-year-old male with a strong alcohol history the alternatives of pancreatic cancer and stomach cancer might be at least temporarily eliminated from the list of active alternatives. This is permissible since these are diseases of older age groups and are not known to be strongly related to alcohol, and urgent intervention is unlikely to affect the outcome of the disease. Eliminating a very unlikely but serious disease from initial active consideration may seem a necessary but dangerous practice. Thus, clinicians must keep these and other serious diseases in the backs of their minds, where they can again be considered if diagnosis or therapy does not go as expected.

## STEP 4. DISEASE: DISEASE IDENTIFICATION BY HYPOTHESIS TESTING

Armed with an initial hypothesis and a differential diagnosis of alternative diseases, clinicians continue to collect data that strengthen or weaken support for their initial hypothesis compared with other diseases in the differential diagnosis. Further data collection may include more extensive history taking, physical examination, or laboratory tests. If further testing does not strengthen the support for the initial hypothesis, the steps can be recycled as the other alternatives are considered.

Hypothesis testing through collection of additional data can be a highly efficient means of distinguishing among the disease possibilities. Disease alternatives can be examined one-by-one against the hypothesized disease, discarding the least likely of each pair until the most likely disease is chosen. In this way diagnostic tests can be conducted or ordered, not to cover all possibilities, but rather as a means of distinguishing between alternative diseases. Tests ordered under conditions of high suspicion usually have the ability to rule in a disease if positive. Tests ordered to rule out an already unlikely possibility are quite reliable in ruling out a disease when they are negative.

A clinician, for instance, might test the hypothesis of duodenal ulcer by having the patient drink some liquid antacids. Rapid relief of the pain would suggest duodenal ulcer or gastritis. For definitive identification of duodenal ulcer, however, an upper gastrointestinal x ray (upper GI) or direct visualization by fiberoptic endoscopy is often needed. To rule out pancreatitis, the clinician might order serum amylase and lipase. By testing to rule in or rule out specific diseases in the active differential, clinicians can more confidently and more efficiently identify the presence of a particular disease.

It is not surprising that George Williams' pain responds rapidly to antacids and that he does have a duodenal ulcer on his upper GI x ray.

## STEP 5. EXPLANATION

The final step in the SHADE process is to determine whether the disease or diseases that have been identified explain some or all the patient's clinical manifestations. This step also represents the clinician's effort to explain whether the disease is due to an underlying cause. Explanation is the final step in diagnosis. By diagnosis, as opposed to disease, we mean the identification of the cause(s), disease(s), and clinical manifestation(s) tied together by an explanation. The full diagnosis may then be diagrammed as follows:

Cause-------------> Disease-------------> Clinical
(alcohol)          (duodenal ulcer)    manifestation
                                       (epigastric pain)

Thus, to completely define a diagnosis we need to establish the existence of three entities:

—Cause
—Disease
—Clinical manifestations

A diagnosis implies more than that these three entities exist in a patient. A diagnosis implies that they fit together and that they have an adequate and coherent explanation. The clinical manifestations are due to the disease, which in turn is preceded by one or more causes that increase the probability that the disease will occur.

This complicated process traditionally has been accomplished relatively simply by utilizing the principle of parsimony. The principle of parsimony states that, if possible the clincian should put together as one disease process the cause, the disease, and the clinical manifestation. Using the principle of parsimony, one disease process is all that is necessary to provide an adequate and coherent explanation of the patient's problem(s).

This final step requires the clinician to mentally step back and attempt to see the whole patient. By recognizing relationships between symptoms, the physician is better able to see the big picture and recognize the diagnosis.

When looking at our patient, George Williams, the physician must ask whether it is possible to provide an adequate and coherent explanation for his problems. When we step back we realize that Mr. Williams not only has clinical manifestations consistent with a duodenal ulcer, he also drinks five to six martinis on weekdays with "a little more" on weekends. Using the principle of parsimony, clinicians often quickly and correctly conclude that one disease process puts together his alcohol, his ulcer, and his epigastric pain.

In applying the SHADE approach to George Williams' problems, we have gone through the following steps:

Symptom: Episodes of pain in the pit of the stomach before meals and awakening at night
Hunch: Duodenal ulcer
Alternatives actively considered: Gastritis, gastric ulcer, pancreatitis
Disease: Duodenal ulcer
Explanation: Alcohol-induced duodenal ulcer producing epigastric pain

As we have seen, the SHADE approach to diagnosis can be a very efficient and practical means of making a diagnosis. It can focus our attention, draw on our knowledge, and build on our analytical skills. It recognizes the limitations of human memory, human attention, and human data-handling ability. As we will see, however, a variety of techniques is necessary to maximize the success of the SHADE process when dealing with more complex clinical problems. In addition, there are inherent limitations of the SHADE process that may lead to medical mistakes.

Scientific study of decision making in medicine has demonstrated the difficult job that confronts us as clinicians. To approach this complicated job, clinicians, like other decision makers, use rules-of-thumb called heuristics. Heuristics intentionally simplify reality, making it possible to deal with the complexities of the world around us.

The SHADE approach is really a collection of rules-of-thumb that together serve to guide the diagnostic process. Those who have studied the heuristics of medical decision making have also identified a parallel set of biases. Biases are predictable problems that occur in the process of decision making and result because the rules-of-thumb are really an over-simplification of reality[1].

Thus if we wish to maximize our diagnostic skills it is necessary to strive for two goals.

1. We need to gain facility utilizing the rules-of-thumb.
2. We need to recognize and learn ways of circumventing the problems inherent in use of these rules-of-thumb.

The relationship between useful heuristics that work well under straightforward situations and the problems that can occur when we apply these heuristics in more complex situations is illustrated by how our eyes and mind estimate distance. When we look at objects at a distance, we use the degree of clarity as a primary rule-of-thumb to help us estimate an object's distance. The clearer an object appears, the closer we estimate its location. This rule-of-thumb often serves us well because in most situations more distant objects are seen less clearly than closer objects. Reliance on this heuristic can lead to serious danger when visibility is poor. When driving down the road on a foggy night, we may dangerously overestimate the distance of an oncoming car. It is hoped that experience has taught us to place less reliance on clarity and more on other cues when driving on a foggy night. Similarly, we need to recognize the limitations of the rules-of-thumb we use in the diagnostic process and learn means to circumvent their problems.

Let us now return to the five steps in the SHADE approach to diagnosis. In each step we will look at the rules-of-thumb, the difficulties in using the rules, and the problems that follow from these rules. Along the way we will look at what we can do to successfully apply these rules-of-thumb and at methods we can use to avoid the consequences of the inherent problems.

# 2

# *Symptoms:*
## *Focusing on a Chief Complaint*

The goal of the first step in the diagnostic process is to identify and accurately characterize the patient's symptoms. We then seek to use the patient's symptoms as a focus or pivot for developing a hunch or disease hypothesis and a list of alternative diseases.

Clinicians frequently use a rapid-focusing process to accomplish this goal. This focusing process is parallel to the way human vision works. We focus in by using our central vision. Once focused, we regard what we're looking at as the relevant field and ignore the background. It is possible to shift from field to background and background to field or back again, but it is not possible to see both at the same time.

Clinicians' reliance on the focusing effect often causes them to rapidly try to take control of the medical interview. In fact, Burack found in a primary-care clinical practice that after an average of 18 seconds of free or open-ended expression by the patient the physician took control. Physicians take control by such expressions as "let me ask you some questions," simply asking yes-no questions or using the physician's favorite expression "OK" followed by a change in subject[2].

The tendency to take control of the medical interview is deep seated in physicians' behavior. Clinicians have traditionally viewed the medical interview much as lawyers have viewed witnesses, even expert witnesses. Clinicians have no question regarding who's in control, who asks the questions, and who has the right to raise objection to the response as out of order or unresponsive to the question.

At first impression taking control appears to increase the physician's efficiency and at times it does. However, from what we know about the focusing effect, we should not be surprised to find that once we focus on a symptom it is hard for us to adjust our initial impression. It is hard for us to see our field as background. Thus, associated with the focusing effect is a bias toward **anchoring** our attention. Anchoring keeps the mind fixed, producing subsequent resistance to change or adjustment. If the patient's initial symptoms turn out to be adequate for the diagnostic process, the anchoring bias doesn't affect the process. However, the process of rapidly focusing on a chief complaint may produce a series of medical mistakes:

Failure to recognize the patient's true purpose for seeking medical care
Failure to clarify conclusion
Failure to maximize and evaluate reliability
Failure to obtain data available through nonverbal communication
Failure to reexamine the original focus

## FAILURE TO RECOGNIZE THE PATIENT'S TRUE PURPOSE

Burack found that nearly half of all patients presenting for medical care had "an underlying motivation other than the presenting complaint." He concluded that the "presenting complaint may bear little resemblance to the principal problem ultimately defined." The presenting symptom may instead serve other functions, including legitimatization of the clinical encounter since patients often feel a need to have a legitimate reason for seeking medical care[2]. In this situation focusing on the chief complaint may prevent discovery of the true reason for the visit.

Perhaps because of the focusing effect and the subsequent physician control of the interview, physicians are frequently frustrated by patients whose true purpose for seeking care is voiced just as the doctor prepares to leave the examining room. It is common to hear a patient state "I guess I should tell you . . . or "You really should know . . . or "I forgot to mention that . . . ." This recurring doorknob syndrome characterizes the patient whose initial symptoms are not a reflection of his or her principal concerns or problem. Perhaps even more frequently the patient's true purpose goes unspoken, and patients leave frustrated despite the physician's best efforts to analyze the presenting complaint.

How can physicians do better? Focusing on the patient's true purpose is often aided when the physician asks or the patient volunteers "why now"? Why has a patient with a complicated, chronic, or confusing history come for care now? What has changed? What really concerns the patient? Understanding "why now" can often uncover the true purpose of the visit and serve as a starting point in pinning down the history.

Another way to get at the reason for the visit and gain additional insight is to ask patients what they fear might be the reason for their problems. At times patients may provide valuable insights, letting you know that they're worried about exposure to AIDS, a chemical at work, or the side effects of their medication. Alternatively, they may alert you to their rational or irrational fears. The fact that their father died of rectal cancer at age 60 and that next month they'll turn 60 may alert you to real risks as well as anxieties that need to be addressed. Occasionally, asking patients what they think is producing their symptoms may be the trigger for a whole new focus of questioning; for instance, when the patient responds "it's that voice that keeps telling me to do it."

Many times it is not obvious why patients come to see a doctor. The existence of symptoms is not enough. It has been estimated that Americans experience a symptom every six days on average, yet they visit physicians only once every few months[3]. Conversely, many persons who do visit doctors do not have progressive medical conditions. Thus, hidden agendas and hidden fears often must be uncovered. When trying to explain why a patient presents for medical care Young suggests using the mnemonic COME[4].

**C**hronic conditions: Patients see physicians for doctor-initiated follow-up, reevaluation and refills.

**O**pinions: Patients see physicians for advice and increasingly often for second opinions.

**M**ild: When the symptoms seem mild—at least from the doctor's perspective—hidden agendas are often at work. These include a need to confide or confess or the fear of a dread disease.

**E**xamination: Routine examination as part of prevention is becoming increasingly common, but an examination may be triggered by administrative or legal needs as well as the same hidden agendas that bring patients in for mild symptoms.

Understanding why patients seek medical care often requires that the physician get the big picture. The importance of getting the big picture has long been recognized by radiologists. It has become standard procedure for radiologists to stand back and take a look at the whole film before focusing in too fast. Looking at the obvious finding last has become an important rule in radiology.

Getting the big picture and the patient's true purpose often require clinicians to give up a little control. Clinicians need to let patients have their say. As Enslaw and Swisher write: "Spontaneous reporting tends to produce the broadest range of information, most of which is likely to be relevant . . ."[5]. Instead of "OK" meaning "let me ask the questions," clinicians can facilitate the patient's discussion by a nod of the head, a supportive "mmm, mmm" or a non-interpretative "yes" or "I see." Even an "I don't follow you" or "I'm sorry but I'm not sure I understand" can encourage the patient to go on to clearly present his or her perception of the problem. When a more vivid description is sought a clinician might ask the patient to describe the problem "so I can picture it happening to me." Facilitation and channeling the patient's own account of the history are more than a means to make patients feel like they're being listened to. Albert writes, "It is vastly more efficient to narrow the diagnostic possibilities by the patient's account than by the clinician's questioning. If we had to enumerate all the possible causes of a cough and all their different manifestations and ask the patient about each one, we would be in for a long night indeed. Simply letting the patient recount the problem usually provides sufficient information to narrow the field immensely in a short time"[6].

It is often ideal to get the big picture at the beginning before focusing too fast. However, all is not lost if the physician can sit back at the end of the interview and ask, as Philip Tumulty advises in his classic book *The Effective Clinician*, "Now is there anything else you want to tell me about yourself or your illness?"[7]

## FAILURE TO CLARIFY CONFUSION

In addition to identifying the patient's symptoms and reasons for seeking care, the physician must accurately characterize these symptoms. Just as radiologists stress the quality of the film, the clinician must ensure the clarity and reliability of the data. Physicians need to accurately understand the nature of a patient's symptoms. An accurate understanding often requires asking specific questions that pin down the meaning of the patient's words. Confusion occurs in history taking because physicians and patients often differ in what they mean by words and what they mean by concepts. Detailed history taking is often required to be sure of the meaning. For instance, in questioning George Williams we would want to know about blood in the stool, vomiting blood, and diarrhea. These are common terms with important implications that require clarification.

When asked whether they have blood in the stool, most patients will respond "yes" only if they note red blood. Few patients have the medical knowledge to recognize black, tarry stools as containing blood. Likewise, most patients will realize they are vomiting blood only if the color is red. The appearance of coffee-grounds in vomit that is characteristic of hematemesis, or vomited blood exposed to stomach acid, is often totally unfamiliar to patients.

Diarrhea is a poorly defined term that has different meaning for different patients. At one extreme, watery stools may not represent diarrhea to patients because no stool is present. At the other extreme, patients may equate one soft stool a day with diarrhea. The physician, with the patient's help, needs to clarify the symptoms to determine whether they truly constitute a problem.

Patients often attempt to assist physicians by using diagnostic terms to communicate the history. The patient may say, "I have a sinus infection" or "I have a migraine headache." It is helpful to know what the patient thinks is wrong, but this should not substitute for a specific description of the symptoms.

Clinicians may add further confusion when they fail to appreciate what their words mean to patients. "Do you take any medications?" may mean to the patient, "Has a doctor prescribed any medications?" Aspirin, vitamins, or a myriad of other over-the-counter medications may escape detection.

The clarity of a patient's history is often improved by efforts to assist the patient to locate and quantitate the symptoms. Efforts to point to the maximum point of pain with one finger often helps in localization. Patients can also be assisted in providing precise quantitation of symptoms. Symptoms that change over time can be measured by asking patients "if 10 is usual for you, and you were 0 when the symptoms were at their peak, where are you now?"

Clinicians' and patients' efforts to measure their degree of symptoms often result in summary descriptions such as "frequently," "usually," "commonly," or "seldom." Investigators have found that these terms have very different meanings to different patients and different doctors. Worse are the double negatives "not uncommon," "not infrequent," and "not unusual." These have been shown to mean more than 75 percent of the time to some and less than 25 percent of the time to others.[8] History taking requires and deserves greater precision on the part of doctors and patients.

## FAILURE TO MAXIMIZE AND EVALUATE RELIABILITY

In order to obtain an accurate account of the symptoms, clinicians must also assess the reliability of the patient's history and, if necessary, obtain alternative sources of accurate information. When evaluating reliability, clinicians need to recognize that patients' past experience may unconsciously alter their perception of the current symptoms. Individuals, for instance, often interpret pain in light of their past experience. A patient with a history of a gallbladder attack may perceive his or her symptoms as identical to the previous gallbladder attack, while actually experiencing a myocardial infarction.

In order to elevate reliability, physicians should also recognize and assess the degree to which a patient is suggestible. Some patients will consciously or unconsciously provide answers they believe their physician wants. To assess this tendency, physicians can ask questions that suggest the reverse of the expected answer. While gently moving a potentially painful joint or examining a painful abdomen, a clinician might ask "does this make the pain better?" A response such as "No, that makes it worse" can then be taken as a reliable answer.

At times it is best to recognize the limits of language and proceed to other techniques for gathering data. These techniques need not involve high-powered technology. Information can often be obtained from patients by nonverbal means. For instance, a patient struggling to describe a change in heart rhythm can often tap out with one finger the speed and pattern of the arrythmia even if he or she can't describe it in words. Dizziness can result from disease in several systems, each with its own special set of symptoms. Verbally distinguishing these forms of dizziness may be very difficult for patients. However, patients can often provide important information if they are asked whether their symptoms are reproduced during a series of maneuvers such as rotating in a chair, quickly standing up, or hyperventilating.

Patients who recognize their own difficulty in describing the symptoms can still provide critical data by noting the circumstances that make the symptoms better or worse. Patients often give a more informative history when they keep a diary of symptoms. Those with recurrent episodes can note the preceding events, frequency, duration, location, and associated symptoms when the episode recurs. Patients can also gather important data by performing simple techniques such as timing their pulse, taking antacids, or lying down to test the effect on symptoms. Physicians and patients who recognize the problems inherent in history taking can seek and find creative ways to reliably report and record the symptoms experienced.

At times the history will indicate that the patient is not the optimal source for obtaining a reliable history. For instance, after obtaining the patient's permission, the patient's family or professional colleagues may help in distinguishing between depression, senility, and drug abuse. Recognition of nighttime hypoglycemia may require a family's help in obtaining a history of sleep walking, restlessness, or other unusual behavior. Just as it is important to know when to obtain secondary sources, it is important to know when the patient's account of the history is critical. Telephone calls can be especially dangerous. Except in dire emergencies or severe language barriers, phone conversations with friends or relatives should not totally replace discussion with the patient. The family who calls because the patient is "not available" or "too sick" to talk offers ominous opportunities for error. Doctors and patients need to recognize that telephone medicine is difficult enough when talking to the patient; it can be treacherous when dealing second hand.

Obtaining the optimal source of data may be critical when a patient has been previously identified as having a disease. Before accepting and perpetuating the existence of an important disease, the current physician should evaluate the data. Patients may be able to identify the types of tests that were obtained and may relate what they were told about the results. Patients, however, cannot be expected to know or remember all the necessary data. The patient's records are often the best source for documenting the previous diseases and for assessing the certainty or uncertainty that existed. For instance, a "heart attack" could actually have been pericarditis or an arrhythmia. "Colitis" may mean spastic colon, ulcerative colitis, or a self-limiting diarrhea. Obtaining the old records or talking to the previous physician may provide information unobtainable in any other way.

Finally, reliability can be increased by using a systemic method for being sure that all essential areas are covered. To maximize the reliability of data that comes from an x ray film, radiologists use a systematic scanning process when reading an x ray. By looking at the same parts of the x ray in the same order each time, they not only can avoid premature focusing, but they can be sure that no area of important data has been missed. Clinicians frequently use the review of symptoms to achieve this benefit of scanning. Asking the same questions in the same order does help to be sure that the critical bases have been covered.

## FAILURE TO OBTAIN THE DATA ACCESSIBLE THROUGH NONVERBAL COMMUNICATION

Focusing too quickly on the patient's chief complaint may keep us from obtaining other essential data. A common error in history taking is to ignore the data that is immediately available from observation of the patient's body language. Human communication is under varying degrees of conscious control. Verbal communication is the focus of much of our conscious mental efforts. However, it reveals to the world what we want known or believe we can safely reveal. Verbal communication may be susceptible to the "Freudian slip" revealing our underlying feelings, doubts, or fears. Verbal communication, however, is governed by a variety of social inhibitions that may prevent a patient from fully revealing inner emotions, the whole story, or true attitudes.

Nonverbal communication on the other hand is to a varying degree under less conscious control. Nonverbal communication comes from a variety of sources including:

Autonomic responses
Body positions
Hand gestures and facial expressions

Desmond has ranked these sources of body language in this order on a Believability Scale[9]. The less-conscious control that can be exerted over body language, the more likely it is to reveal inner thoughts or emotions. Let us examine these modes of nonverbal communication starting with those farthest removed from conscious control.

Autonomic responses—sweating, blushing, breathing, and pupillary responses—are examples of autonomic signals that are difficult to control consciously. The sweaty palms of anxiety and the facial or body blush of embarrassment are communications whose reliability is very high. Breathing patterns often reveal underlying mood or emotions. The sigh of relief when learning that a symptom is not cancer and the periodic sigh of anxiety or depression are revealing gestures of underlying emotions.

Body posture is a time-honored clinical means of assessing underlying attitude and mood. The slumping posture of dejection or depression is an important clinical cue. Crossed arms and leaned-back posture suggest defensiveness or suspicion. Leaning forward signals attention or excitement, while slumping reveals boredom or disinterest. Body posturing, however, often comes under conscious control, and patients frequently try to position themselves to express interest or attention to a physician. Withdrawn, dejected, or slumping postures are thus even more revealing if they occur when attention and interest would usually be expected.

Most individuals use hand gestures and facial expressions to reinforce their verbal expressions. We all use facial expressions constantly to judge the intensity of symptoms and emotions. As clinicians we tend to judge the severity of pain by the patient's grimacing gesture, and the degree of fear and anxiety is judged by the anxious or worried look on the patient's face. Yet the hands and face are under greater conscious control so we can be fooled. Hand gestures and facial expressions are learned behavior whose reliability is less certain than other gestures. When the face and hands concur with the words we are often impressed, but when they concur with the rest of the body language, we can gain even greater confidence. As an old Chinese proberb says, "Watch out for the man whose stomach doesn't move when he laughs."

Facial expressions are so much a part of our everyday communication that the absence of intricate expressions should raise suspicions of serious underlying disease. Parkinsonism due to either drugs or disease is characterized by decreased facial expression. The less animated countenance may also suggest depression.

Attention to body language helps to ensure that we have not missed important cues. It also helps confirm the quality and reliability of our data. Reading the patient's body language is a skill that isn't likely to be replaced by a computer. Knowing its nuances is essential to quality care.

## FAILURE TO REEXAMINE THE ORIGINAL FOCUS

In the first step in the SHADE approach to diagnosis we focus on a chief complaint, aiming to recognize the patient's true purpose, clarify confusion, rate reliability, and obtain data available through verbal and nonverbal communication. At times, however, the process of rapidly focusing can lead us down a blind alley by anchoring our thought process on an unproductive approach. Thus, it is essential that clinicians learn how to switch gears and get out of these blind alleys. We must learn to step back and refocus. Clinicians frequently try to define a patient's chief complaint hoping to determine the most productive symptom to use as the focus or pivot for the diagnostic process. At times, however, the patient's chief complaint may not serve as a useful focus for the diagnostic process.

Patients, for instance, may present with problems such as nausea, fatigue, or nervousness. These symptoms may not serve as a useful focus for the diagnostic process since they are difficult to characterize reliably, have nearly unlimited alternatives, and can be due to a variety of pathophysiologic processes. In contrast, epigastric pain, weight loss, or tremor are more definite, have limited differential probabilities, and are often explained by a basic pathophysiologic process.

The difficulty of dealing with vague complaints, however, often encourages physicians to focus on objective signs and symptoms suggestive of organic disease. This tendency can be partially overcome if physicians seek positive evidence and objective symptoms of emotional disorders, and emphasize clusters of symptoms consistent with anxiety, depression, and psychoses. Sleep disturbances, thought disturbances, and evidence of physical and social withdrawal can be as effective a focus for the diagnostic process as jaundice, blood in the stool, or a third nerve palsy.

At times vague and unlimited symptoms must by necessity serve as the basis for hypothesis formation and differential diagnosis. They may even be the only symptoms. Often, however, physicians are confronted by a series of symptoms, a chief complaint, plus a variety of associated symptoms. At these times it is useful to evaluate which symptoms to use as the basis for hypothesis formation and differential diagnosis. Confronted with a chief complaint of nausea the focal point might be better directed at the associated weight loss, jaundice, or missed menses. Faced with a chief complaint of headache the associated symptoms of hearing loss, arm weakness, or purulent nasal discharge may be a more efficient focus for the work-up.

The choice of which symptom to use as the focus or pivot for hypothesis generation is often crucial. Thus the symptom chosen as the pivot or focus determines which is field and which is background. The symptom chosen as the pivot or focus helps determine the answer we obtain. Fever and a new heart murmur, for instance, rapidly leads to consider endocarditis, while using pleuritic chest pain as the focus may put endocarditis out of primary consideration. Similarly, in a patient with back pain and claudication framing the question as one of back pain may make the consideration of aortic aneurysm less obvious than if one actively considers the differential of claudication. Astute clinicians can reach the same diagnosis through both routes, but efficient and timely diagnosis is easier if care is taken in selecting which symptom(s) to use as the focus. When in doubt, it is often best to try multiple combinations since each combination may bring to mind a different hypothesis. There is no rule that says a patient should have only one complaint or a physician should have only one hypothesis.

While selecting a chief complaint, ensuring clear and reliable data, getting the big picture, and refocusing if necessary, it is hoped that we are doing more than collecting information. We are thinking about the information to generate an early hunch or hypothesis. Thus, let us turn to the second step in the diagnostic process: generating an early hypothesis.

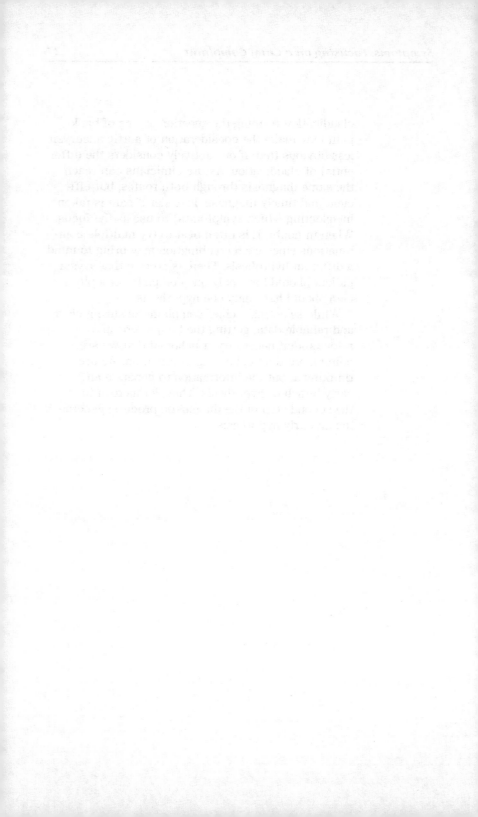

# *3*

# *Hunches:*
## *Generating an Early Hypothesis*

The process of hypothesis formation is a natural and early outgrowth of the process of focusing on a chief complaint. In medical practice disease hypotheses are often rapidly generated by matching the patient's symptoms with those of the classic or textbook description of a disease. This matching process utilizes a rule-of-thumb or heuristic known as the *representativeness heuristic*. Representativeness implies that we naturally have hunches that are brought to mind by the degree to which the patient's symptoms match up with the classic patterns of disease that are stored in our memory. Often this matching process works well and expedites the process of hypothesis formation. When the pattern fits well, efficient and successful disease identification usually occurs. The acquisition of knowledge of disease patterns or schema constitutes much of what is learned in medical education and in later training and experience. Classic patterns of disease are formally taught in medical school. One can think of those patterns of disease as trees. Students learn about the trunks and their major branches. Years of training and experience provide the twigs and the leaves.

For students beginning clinical medicine, the problem may be the lack of knowledge of the classic pattern. For most well-trained clinicians, this problem is soon overcome and the challenge is to make more sophisticated use of pattern matching, utilizing the representativeness heuristic. Despite the usefulness of the representativeness rule-of-thumb, it is important to recognize that it may lead clinicians to jump to conclusions. Clinicians can learn to avoid jumping to conclusions by listing the patient's symptoms or problems in a problem list before proceeding to combine them. Clinicians can also consciously focus on a broad hypothesis such as cardiac disease, cerebral vascular disease, or infection rather than jumping to a narrow hypothesis such as coronary artery disease, vascular malfunction, or cryptococcal meningitis.

Both students and experienced clinicians must struggle with some basic limitations of pattern matching:

Patients may present with incomplete or modified disease manifestations.
The relevant disease pattern may not be readily brought to mind by the clinician.
Patients may engage in denial and fail to readily and openly convey the critical elements of the pattern.

Each of these explanations creates its own type of barrier to hypothesis generation and requires its own means for minimizing its impact.

## INCOMPLETE OR MODIFIED DISEASE PATTERN

Classic patterns of a disease, the textbook description, are more often a composite of frequent clinical features rather than a pattern that is likely to be totally reproduced in any one patient. Few patients with mononucleosis will have all the classic symptoms of pharnygitis, splenomegaly, lymphadenopathy, and elevated liver enzymes. Few patients with secondary syphilis will have all the possible skin, hair, and lymph node changes, much less the myriad of systemic inflammatory manifestations that help make syphilis a great masquerader.

Presentations with classic patterns of disease are increasingly becoming the exception rather than the rule. Classic descriptions have often been derived from observations of far-advanced or severe disease. Today, patients frequently seek medical care at an early stage in their disease process. Since patients increasingly present for care at an early stage of their disease, they are seen by a physician before their full potential disease pattern has emerged. Clinicians must have a high index of suspicion for bacterial endocarditis even before the appearance of splenomegaly, Roth spots, or the Osler's nodes that are found in only a small percentage of patients with endocarditis. In fact, a patient with endocarditis due to IV drug abuse will often present without even a murmur. Similarly, the clinician who waits for the skin, voice, or hair changes of hypothyroidism will miss the disease in the vast majority of patients.

In addition, with the aging of the population and the proliferation of therapeutic interventions, it is increasingly common to see patients with complicated manifestations or symptoms produced by one disease being modified by other diseases or by the patients' treatment. For instance, control of hypertension may occur as a result of a recognized, or even a silent, myocardial infarction. Patients being treated for hypertension with beta blockers may not demonstrate tachycardia, nervousness, or tremor if they should develop hyperthyroidism.

## BRINGING THE RELEVANT PATTERN TO MIND

In addition to complicated or incomplete disease manifestations, a disease may not be recognized because physicians can't bring the pattern to mind. At times, physicians as well as medical students may simply be unaware of the classic pattern of the disease. Even when this is not the problem, bringing the pattern to mind often requires more than having heard of the classic pattern once. Ease of retrieval requires repeated use. We gain facility in retrieving and manipulating patterns through constant practice. Lack of experience or lack of recent reinforcement using these patterns represents a substantial barrier to retrieval.

Subspecialists often become especially adept at recognizing patterns within their discipline. However, specialists in one area of medicine often have difficulty recognizing diseases outside their field of expertise. Even with repeated use there are several barriers that keep us from making a match between the pattern stored in our memory and the patient's symptoms.

**Everyone has a tendency to see what he or she is looking for and hear what he or she is listening for.** Observation is by no means an objective process. In recent years it has been realized that the commonly occurring heart sound appropriately known as a click is indicative of mitral valve prolapse. These clicks characteristic of mitral valve prolapse may be present in over five percent of otherwise healthy young women. Despite their frequent presence, few clinicians recognized their existence prior to the development of echocardiography, and the widespread efforts to recognize and document their presence. The need to specifically look and listen is compounded by the fact that human beings are distracted by the dramatic and may not see the mundane. Dramatic findings naturally catch one's attention. By focusing on the dramatic, important details outside the central focus of our attention can be missed. For instance, when an injured patient comes to the emergency room with obvious bleeding, the existence of ineffective breathing due to multiple rib fractures may not be immediately noticed. An awareness and a calm systematic search for the less obvious and important clinical findings is required in order to avoid serious consequences.

**We don't see what we don't want to see.** The tendency to avoid recognition of the unpleasant is a human trait that does not spare physicians. Prior to widespread publicity, most physicians rarely recognized child abuse or spouse abuse. The widespread presence of alcohol and drug abuse is still often missed by physicians who do not specifically focus on the subject.

Physicians who do not want to know certain facts often give patients nonverbal or subtle verbal messages that communicate their attitudes. Physicians who are antagonistic to homosexuality rarely hear of it from their patients. Physicians who feel uncomfortable discussing sexuality rarely recognize or are told of impotence by their patients. Physicians see what they want to see, don't see what they don't want to see, and are told what patients think they are willing to hear. The use of routine questions regarding such sensitive subjects as homosexuality, alcohol consumption, and drug abuse helps circumvent this barrier. Once at ease with asking these questions, clinicians are less likely to suppress these important areas of data collection. When the situation is potentially uncomfortable, the clinician may then merely state, "Let me ask you some routine questions."

**Familiarity can cloud our vision.** Familiarity can cloud or distort what all of us hear and see. A physician's friends, relatives, and professional colleagues often seek diagnosis and treatment. The physician's difficulty in being objective can be great. The physician's tendency to treat these individuals differently can be disastrous. It may be hard to ask a colleague about alcohol or drug abuse, a relative about venereal disease or homosexuality, a friend about child abuse or senility. Often the physician doesn't even get a chance to ask these questions because advice is requested or given "off the cuff" as a "curbside consult." Such easy access and casual opinions often do not result in quality medical care.

## DENIAL OF THE CRITICAL ELEMENTS OF THE PATTERNS

In addition to the problems created by complex or incomplete presentations and the barriers to pattern matching, a third source of difficulty preventing disease recognition is the patient's denial. Most of the time patients readily and openly convey the critical elements necessary for the recognition of the disease pattern. Patients, however, may practice unconscious forms of denial that make it difficult for them to recognize and convey critical pieces of medical information.

Denial can occur when patients fail to acknowledge to themselves or to others the existence of a symptom. When patients unconsciously deny symptoms even to themselves they often suspect a severe disease. This type of denial may result in an altered history. A changing mole that has been ignored may be represented by the patient as a sudden growth.

Chest pressure on exertion suggestive of heart disease may not be mentioned, or may be attributed to overexertion. Changes in bowel habits may be ascribed to poor eating habits. These, and many other believable histories, can confuse the physician who is not aware of, or does not allow, for the human tendency for denial. Physicians can often suspect this form of denial by recognizing a patient's fear of disability, surgery, or death.

Denial may take the subtle form of accommodation as patients slowly and semiconsciously adjust to the limitations imposed by their slowly progressive disease. Patients with heart or lung symptoms may reduce their activities and believe their attacks of pain or shortness of breath are the same as they have been. An effort to compare their current and former activity level may uncover this form of denial. Often, however, family and friends recognize these changes even when they are not apparent to the patient.

At times, patients are aware of more than they feel free to express. Fear of social stigma or exposure of personal failure may prevent patients from telling the physician all they know. The subject matter should often alert the physician to the possibility of social denial. Sexually transmitted disease, alcoholism, and drug abuse are all areas in which social denial is common because of the accompanying social stigma. More subtle social denial may occur with hearing loss because of the associated image of growing old. The perception of personal failure may make full disclosure difficult for patients. Tuberculosis still carries for many the connotation of poor hygiene. Likewise, nutritional deficits may be denied by those who cannot afford a balanced diet.

Clinicians must recognize the frequent occurrence of denial if they are to successfully formulate hypotheses. Fortunately, patients are usually willing to trust physicians with even their best-kept secrets if they understand the importance of the questions to their care and the confidentiality of the information. Patients can legitimately expect physicians to be nonjudgmental in addressing sensitive areas of the history. Direct questions are essential, but clinicians must avoid emotionally laden words. "Have you ever used illegal drugs?", "Do you have an alcohol problem?", or "is he a good boy or a problem child?" rarely produce open communication. Clinicians who put the patient on the defensive by their questioning should expect this patient to look elsewhere for a more sympathetic ear.

We have now examined the barriers to producing hunches or hypotheses, including complex or incomplete disease manifestation, barriers to pattern matching, and denial. We have also suggested methods for physicians to circumvent these problems. Let us now turn to the next step in the diagnostic process, developing a differential diagnosis.

# 4

# *Alternatives:*
## *Developing a Differential Diagnosis*

Once a hunch or hypothesis has been formulated, clinicians often recognize the existence of a list of alternative disease possibilities. The limited ability of human beings to actively consider large numbers of alternatives, and the increasing cost of testing for all the possibilities, require physicians to weigh the possibilities and come up with a limited list of alternatives for active consideration.

In developing this differential diagnosis, the goal is different than in hypothesis formation. In hypothesis formation, the clinician seeks to produce a probable-disease hypothesis. In contrast, in forming a differential diagnosis the clinician seeks to think of all reasonable and important disease entities and retain a selected and limited list for active consideration.

Clinicians tend to use a rule-of-thumb known as
the availability heuristic, when developing a differential diagnosis. Availability means what comes easily to mind. The clinician can often bring to mind
many more possibilities by systematically searching
his or her memory, than by casual consideration of
those diseases that come easily to mind. Physicians
can enhance the use of the availability heuristic by
proceeding through a formal process of searching
their memory. Often this is facilitated by thinking
through categories of disease. Disease can be organized by mechanisms such as infectious, metabolic,
cancer, collagen-vascular, and iatrogenic. In addition, thinking through such a list brings to mind
sublists. Having thought through diseases by mechanism, a second search by organ symptom may bring
other possibilities to mind. A third search, using
clinical checklists based on the patient's problems,
such as hematuria, vertigo, or edema, may bring to
mind still further possibilities.

Clinicians who utilize computerized, diagnostic
aids often are impressed by the number of possibilities that the computer can retrieve—often many
that are totally inappropriate and can be easily
dismissed. Yet among these long lists of irrelevent
diseases there are often one or two that don't seem
so ridiculous and need to be considered. Often the
clinician will say, "How come I didn't think of
that . . . I know about it." The human mind, like the
computer, can and does store an enormous quantity
of disease information. The problem is often orga-
nizing and accessing that information. It is important for clinicians to be aware of how their medical
education has organized the input so they can use
these frameworks to search their memories and
obtain the needed output. Practice using systematic
searches employing more than one framework
can help clinicians access their own mental
computers.

There are a number of types of mistakes that are made by relying exclusively on the availability heuristic when selecting diseases to include in the active list of alternatives:

Failure to consider disease known to present with misleading manifestations due to medical mirages or masquerades.

Failure to consider common disease presenting with unusual features

Looking for rare disease or zebras without a good reason

## MEDICAL MIRAGES AND MASQUERADES

Certain diseases with a propensity to present in a misleading fashion can create diagnostic blind spots. These diseases frequently present as medical mirages or masquerades. Medical mirage occurs when symptoms perceived by the patient in one area or organ system actually originate in another location or system. Medical masquerades occur when a disease presents with symptoms and signs that suggest a different disease.

Medical mirages are frequently the result of referred symptoms. Referred symptoms may be the result of changes in position of the heart, esophagus, larynx, or thyroid that occur as part of embryonic development. Thus, pain originating in the heart and esophagus may be felt by the patient in the left arm; while pathology originating in the larynx and thyroid may present as referred symptoms in the throat and ears. Alternatively, symptoms may be referred along the course of peripheral nerves, explaining why leg pain occurs with disc disease, and arm pain may result from nerve compression at the level of the neck.

Certain diseases have gained renown as great masqueraders, presenting in multiple guises easily confused with other diseases. Clinicians must have a knowledge of these conditions and a high index of suspicion to unmask the disease. It is helpful to have a list in the back of your mind of serious treatable disease that often lead clinicians astray. Syphilis has long been called the great masquerader. A variety of other diseases, including, most recently, Acquired Immune Deficiency Syndrome (AIDS), and Lyme disease, rival syphilis in their ability to deceive the unsuspecting clinician. Subacute bacterial endocarditis, miliary tuberculosis, aortic aneurysm, ectopic pregnancy, and pulmonary emboli are other classic masqueraders whose recognition is important.

Recognition of the existence of medical mirages and medical masquerades, plus an explicit effort to include these diseases in the differential diagnosis, can reduce the likelihood that they will deceive the clinician.

## COMMON DISEASE PRESENTING WITH UNUSUAL FEATURES

It is also important to take into account the prevalence or frequency of the disease when deciding which diseases to include in the active list of alternatives. The bias known as "ignoring the base-rate effect", means that physicians tend to rely on how well the patterns match, rather than how frequently the disease occurs.

An old clinical pearl states that "Common disease occurs commonly." This is true even when they appear with uncommon clinical manifestations not included in their classic pattern. The occurrence of atypical symptoms is so frequent as to justify another clinical maxim, "Atypical presentations of common diseases are more frequent than the classical presentation of rare diseases." Thus the frequency of a disease deserves overt recognition in the process of creating an active differential diagnosis. Because of its frequency of occurrence, duodenal ulcer must be considered even when the abdominal pain is not classic for duodenal ulcer. Alcohol-induced symptoms deserve consideration even when alcohol is not obviously implicated. Myocardial infarction deserves consideration whenever pain presents from "the nose to the navel." In fact if George Williams had been 50 years old with risk factors for coronary artery disease, myocardial infarction should have been included among the alternatives for the pain in the pit of his stomach. Myocardial infarction also should enter into the differential diagnosis of such symptoms as dizziness, shortness of breath, and unexplained fatigue.

The baseline frequency or prevalence of a disease is most easily included in our consideration if we ask "Is this the right setting or the right type of patient?" We are trying to determine not only how common a disease is, but how common the disease is in a particular type of patient. It's not enough to know that lung cancer and chronic-obstructive lung disease are common diseases; we must recognize that they increase with age and cigarette smoking. Thus, in a 60-year-old chronic smoker these diseases should be high on the differential list even when the pattern of symptoms doesn't match the expected pattern.

## LOOKING FOR ZEBRAS WITHOUT GOOD REASON

"When you hear hoofbeats, it is more likely a horse than a zebra," goes the clinical wisdom. Yet identifying the zebra has provided great intellectual satisfaction to many physicians. The search for the rare disease, however, may keep clinicians from seeing the obvious. In medicine we overlook the obvious at our own peril and that of the patient. In a cost-conscious era it is no longer possible to pursue every zebra. The detection of rare diseases, however, is still an important role for physicians. Knowing when and how to look for the rare disease can be critically important. Let us outline a series of good reasons to consider a rare disease in the active differential diagnosis.

## When the Consequences Can Be Contained

With some rare diseases the natural history can be altered by early therapy. These diseases deserve special consideration and investigation. Unilateral hearing loss should bring to mind acoustic neuroma and cholesteatoma. These conditions can be successfully treated, especially when early intervention occurs. Diagnosing other treatable zebras involves only minor modification of the usual diagnostic steps. When working-up unexplained elevations in liver function tests, Wilson's disease and hemochomatosis should be included in the active differential diagnosis since their identification is safe, relatively economical, and their treatment is effective if begun early.

## When the Case is Complex

While most complex clinical situations involve multiple diseases, there are a number of rare diseases whose diagnosis can help to explain apparently unrelated symptoms. These diseases are often worth remembering and pursuing since they help avoid multiple invasive investigations, and help to guide overall therapy. The diagnosis of acromegaly may explain hyperglycemia, arthritis, headaches, and amenorrhea. The pursuit of Addison's disease may be life saving in the setting of hypotension, hypothermia, and sepsis. The diagnosis of polyarteritis nodosum may lead to better therapy for hypertension, neurological symptoms, and renal disease. The existence of unexplained symptoms in several organ systems should trigger the search for rare diseases.

## When the Answer is Elusive

Having worked-up a patient without producing a satisfactory diagnosis, one should begin to reconsider the likelihood of an unusual disease. When right-sided heart failure is present in the absence of pulmonary disease or chronic pulmonary emboli, constrictive pericarditis should be investigated. When shoulder pain cannot be explained by the usual intrinsic neck or shoulder pathology, pancoast tumors in the apex of the lung should be considered along with other diseases of the chest. The likelihood of rare disease becomes greater when there is no evidence to support the more-common disease. Therefore, when common disease has been excluded, but signs or symptoms persist, it is reasonable to think of rare diseases.

## When the Pattern Suggests Something Unusual

Another reason for pursuing rare disease is when the pattern suggests that the patient's problems are different from the expected. Experienced clinicians often are able to utilize the representativeness heuristic to sense that something doesn't fit just right. This sixth sense is really their ability to know disease patterns well enough to sense when the usual disease doesn't fit. The occurrence of unilateral wheezing should initiate a search for an obstructive lesion. The occurrence of urinary infections in males should alert the physician to possible underlying pathology. Usually those hoofbeats are more likely to be a horse than a zebra, but it depends where you are. What is rare in one setting is common in another. AIDS has made diseases once regarded as zebras all too commonplace. Thus it is important to look for a zebra when the pattern suggests something unusual.

Experienced physicians can usually retrieve a long list of potential alternatives, far longer than can efficiently be evaluated. Thus, the more difficult step in this process is to determine which diseases to include in the active differential diagnosis, that is, the diseases that will be ruled in or ruled out by testing.

In assessing which diseases to include in the active differential diagnosis, it is often helpful to list the pros and cons for each possibility. In George Williams' case, for instance, pancreatitis was favored because of his alcohol history, but the intermittent nature of the symptoms were against the presence of pancreatitis. The evidence for pancreatitis was strong enough to include it in the active differential diagnosis and to use serum amylase and lipase to rule it out. Where there are more than one or two symptoms and multiple disease possibilities, it is helpful to write down a list of disease manifestations and disease alternatives. Then it is possible to ask which of the disease manifestations can be explained by each of the diseases. "Without access to a list of those symptoms that actually did and did not occur,"[9] writes Arkes, "one tends to remember the facts supportive of the hypothesis under consideration and to forget the facts inconsistent with the hypothesis."[10]

The effort to use the data to support or refute each possibility means that diseases will not need to be identified by exclusion. Even psychiatric diseases, for which there are few high-tech diagnostic tests, can be evaluated weighing the evidence for and against the presence of the disease. In deciding which diseases to include in the active differential diagnosis, it is important to remember that using the representativeness heuristic and analyzing how well the clinical manifestations match the pattern of disease is not the only method that should be used. As we will emphasize later in Chapter 7, the urgency and severity of the disease alternative must be considered. Asking, "What's the most life-threatening disease, the patient could have?", is a critical question when thinking through the alternatives and deciding which ones to include in the active differential diagnosis.

Thus, to avoid mistakes in development of a differential diagnosis, clinicians must learn to use the representativeness and availability heuristic. Clinicians, however, must not rely exclusively on these heuristics. Deciding on which diseases to include for active consideration requires that physicians consider:

Common diseases presenting with unusual features
Diseases that are known to present with misleading
    symptoms
Rare disease when we have a good reason

Having developed a hypothesis and a list of alternatives we are now able to proceed to identify a disease.

# 5

# Disease:
## Identification by Hypothesis Testing

Having produced a hypothesis and an active list of alternatives, the clinician's job is to decide between them. The SHADE process requires the clinician to support or refute the hypothesized disease, consider the alternative diseases in the differential diagnosis, and decide between the hypothesis and the alternatives. When testing to achieve disease identification, clinicians rely on what we will call the hypothesis testing heuristic. This rule-of-thumb says that test results, when positive, serve to rule in disease and, when negative, serve to rule out disease. An ideal test would definitively identify a disease if it were positive and definitively rule out a disease if it were negative. This type of test is called a gold-standard test. Gold-standard tests exist for many diseases. Coronary catheterization serves this purpose for coronary artery disease, while biopsy serves as the gold standard for such diseases as hepatic cirrhosis and bronchogenic carcinoma. Unfortunately, they are often too dangerous, too expensive, or otherwise too impractical to use as the initial tests for ruling in or ruling out disease. Thus, the usual tests we use in clinical medicine are less than perfect.

Testing actually begins early in the disease identification process since it is an active part of history taking and physical examination. In fact, history taking has been said to be hypothesis driven since efforts to support or refute a hypothesis often determine the questions that are asked.

Testing of hunches or hypotheses continues as part of the physical examination. Physical examination is actually a collection of diagnostic tests, each of which requires attention to their accuracy of performance, potential false positives, and potential false negatives. A common mistake is to ignore the fact that the physical examination is a collection of diagnostic tests and perform the physical examination by rote, with little thought given to the usefulness of the individual pieces of information obtained. To help avoid this mistake we need to learn how to integrate the physical examination into the diagnostic thought process. Let us start by taking a look at the physical examination as a diagnostic test.

The physical examination has important and unique advantages as a diagnostic test. It offers clinicians a direct method for assessing the patient's ability to function physically, socially, and mentally. The severity of acute gastrointestinal bleeding, the intellectual impairment from Alzheimer's disease, or the functional impairment from hemiparesis or Bell's palsy is best assessed by physical examination, including the mental status examination. Physical examination also offers clinicians the opportunity to perform maneuvers that can add unique diagnostic information. When hypothesizing peritonitis, the clinician can test for rebound tenderness. When hypothesizing meningitis, accentuation of the pain with neck flexion supports the presence of meningitis. Clinicians must also appreciate the limitations of physical examination tests and aim to reduce the inaccuracy, recognize the inherent deficiencies, and use care when interpreting the data. Failure to maximize examination techniques can prevent the collection of meaningful data. A moderately enlarged spleen can only be felt with the patient lying with the left side up. Mild elevation in bilirubin will first be detected in natural light, not under the fluorescent lights of many examining rooms. Inherent inaccuracies in the physical examination need to be recognized. Certain traditional components of the physical examination are of little diagnostic value. Percussion for cardiac size correlates poorly with true heart size. Examination of the knee for ballotment is a very poor method for assessing fluid in the knee. Mere inspection for loss of medial dimpling or alternatively "milking" the fluid into the joint and checking for a fluid wave are much more accurate means of examination.

Patient characteristics may limit the accuracy of the examination or require its modification. Physicians cannot expect to detect abdominal or ovarian masses in obese patients. Pendulous or fibrocystic breasts make examination inherently more difficult. At times the examination can be modified to increase accuracy, such as the use of a larger blood pressure cuff to produce accurate measurements in the obese patient.

When interpreting the physical examination, clinicians must appreciate the common occurrence of normal variants. Normal variants are relatively common stable findings that are easily confused with pathology. As many as five percent of disease-free individuals will have inequality of their pupils, often up to 2 mm on close examination. Their pupils, however, react normally to light. Failure to recognize this normal variation may result in diagnostic confusion when a patient seeks care after a head injury. The normal variant characterized by the absence of optic cupping and even slight blurring of the disc may be confused with increased intercranial pressure. The presence of venous pulsations in this normal variant, however, will distinguish this condition from papilledema.

Finally, when interpreting the physical examination we must take into account the characteristics of the patient. Age, for instance, affects what we expect to observe on physical examination. An S3 is an expected sign in children and young adults, but evidence of pathology in the elderly. Loss of ankle and abdominal reflexes, high-pitched hearing loss, and absence of palpable ovaries are expected findings in the elderly. New benign lesions such as small, bright cherry-red angiomas and waxlike, superficial seborrheic keratoses are very frequent skin changes accompanying aging. Similarly, the development of an isolated S4 or abdominal systolic bruit should raise little concern. When properly performed and interpreted, the physical examination used along with the history can help the physician utilize relatively expensive and potentially dangerous technology. Let us take a look now at the principles we use to assess the usefulness of tests and how failing to understand these principles can lead to medical mistakes.

Once the history and physical examinations are completed and the physician has in hand a hypothesis and a list of active alternatives, diagnostic tests are frequently ordered. A series of medical mistakes can occur in the process of ordering and interpreting diagnostic tests. Let us explore what can go wrong in the process of disease identification by hypothesis testing.

## ORDERING TESTS WITHOUT ASKING WHY

When ordering tests physicians must ask, "Why is the test being ordered?" Tests may be ordered to rule in or rule out disease. When multiple tests exist one test may be used to decide which of two or more invasive tests is best suited to a particular patient. Alternatively, tests may be ordered to decide on the best treatment, to monitor the side effects of therapy, or to assess the response to treatment. One of the most common mistakes clinicians make in using diagnostic tests is failing to address the question "Why is the test being ordered?"

We will now only consider tests that are used as part of diagnosis to rule in or rule out a disease on the differential list. Later in this chapter we will explore mistakes in ordering tests that stem from other justifications used in answering the question "Why is the test being ordered?"

## IMPORTANCE OF ESTIMATING THE PROBABILITY OF DISEASE BEFORE ORDERING TESTS

Having decided to test to rule in or rule out a disease, we need to ask another important question to interpret the results: "What is the probability that the patient has the hypothesized disease before we know the test results?" This may at first seem like an unnecessary waste of time, yet it is critical to making sense of the test results. Let us see why.

To assess the usefulness of clinical tests studies are conducted that compare the clinical test's results with those of the gold standard. Usually these tests agree with the gold-standard result and produce true-positive or true-negative results. However, those clinical tests may disagree with the gold-standard results and produce false-negative and false-positive test results. A false-negative test result occurs when the clinical test is negative but the gold standard test is positive. A false-positive test occurs when the clinical test is positive and the gold-standard test is negative.

The probability of a positive test when disease is present is called the sensitivity. It may be remembered using the mnemonic PID, for "positive in disease." The probability of a negative test in healthy individuals is known as specificity. Thus, specificity may be remembered using the mnemonic NIH, for "negative in health."

For instance, let us imagine that a clinician is evaluating whether a patient has coronary artery disease. Coronary catheterization is the gold-standard test, but clinicians usually perform a safer, less expensive exercise stress test as the initial test when trying to rule in or rule out coronary artery disease. An exercise stress test, however, is a less than perfect test since it produces some false-positive and some false-negative test results when compared to coronary catheterization on the same patient.

If a test has 100 percent sensitivity and 100 percent specificity, it is a perfect test. In this case information about the particular patient's probability of disease before obtaining the test is not necessary. There are very few perfect tests in clinical medicine. The farther the sensitivity and specificity are from 100 percent, the more important the information we have on the patient becomes. In fact, for most clinical tests such as exercise stress testing, the most important factor in interpreting the probability of disease **after** knowing the test results is our best estimate of the probability of disease **before** ordering the test. This probability of disease before ordering a test is known as the pretest probability of disease (or prior probability). Where does this estimate come from? It comes from what we know about the prevalence or frequency of the disease, the patient's risk factors for the disease, and the degree to which the patient's symptoms match the disease pattern.

We know that coronary artery disease is a very common disease, the most common life-threatening disease in the United States. Risk factors that increase the probability of developing and having coronary artery disease include age, elevated cholesterol, high blood pressure, lack of exercise, and smoking cigarettes. Males are at higher risk except among the elderly. In addition, the clinician needs to take into account the symptom patterns of the particular patient and ask whether the patient's symptoms fit the manifestation of coronary artery disease. Thus, when evaluating the probability of coronary artery disease for a 20-year-old female athlete with atypical chest pain without other risk factors for coronary artery disease, the probability of disease is extremely low; a ballpark estimate of one percent or less. In contrast, a 60-year-old man who smokes cigarettes and has recently developed exercise-induced chest pain, typical of the chest pain of coronary artery disease, has a very high probability of the disease; a ballpark estimate of perhaps 50 percent or more. Finally, a 50-year-old woman with high blood pressure who smokes cigarettes and has recently developed shooting chest pain at rest, not typical of coronary artery disease, is at an intermediate risk of disease; a ballpark estimate of perhaps ten percent.

Thus, in developing a probability of disease before ordering a test we need to combine what we know about the prevalence of the disease, the patient's risk factors for the disease, and the degree that the patient's pattern of symptoms matches the disease's pattern. In developing this pretest probability of disease, clinicians usually do not use precise numbers; rather we use estimates like those just discussed.

For illustration, let us assume that before performing the test these three patients had a pretest probability of disease of 1 percent, 50 percent, and 10 percent, respectively. Now imagine that we have performed an exercise stress test and obtained the same positive test on each of these three patients. We will assume that the exercise stress test is a rather good test by clinical standards, having a sensitivity of 90 percent and a specificity of 95 percent.* After having obtained the positive exercise stress test the approximate probabilities of coronary artery disease are:[†]

| | 1% pretest probability of disease | | 10% pretest probability of disease | | 50% pretest probability of disease | |
|---|---|---|---|---|---|---|
| | D (+) | D (−) | D (+) | D (−) | D (+) | D (−) |
| Test + | 9 | 49.5 | 90 | 45 | 450 | 25 |
| Test − | 1 | 940.5 | 10 | 855 | 50 | 475 |
| | 10 | 990 | 100 | 900 | 500 | 500 |

Probability post test

$$\frac{9}{9 + 49.5} = 15\% \qquad \frac{90}{90 + 45} = 67\% \qquad \frac{450}{450 + 25} = 95\%$$

For the 20-year-old female athelete: 15%
For the 60-year-old man with exertional chest pain: 95%
For the 50-year-old woman with atypical chest symptom: 67%

*It is important to recognize that a stress test itself may not be unequivocally positive or negative. Clear cut positive and negative results occur, but there are many equivocal findings in between.

†These probabilities are calculated as follows: The probability of a disease before a test can be used as the prevalence of the disease. Assuming a group of 1000 individuals, the sensitivity and specificity are used to fill in the following 2 × 2 tables.

Thus, the probability of disease after obtaining the result of a test—the posttest probability—is often dramatically affected by our best ballpark estimate of the pretest probability of the disease. To successfully use positive tests to rule in disease and negative tests to rule out disease we need to pay attention to the pretest probability of disease.

Once a test is ordered problems exist in interpreting its results. These problems include:

Failure to fully utilize negative test results
Failure to recognize the limitations of positive and
  negative test results defined by a range of normal
Overreliance on the weight of the evidence and
  susceptibility to information overload when
  combining test results

## Utilizing Negative Test Results

The hypothesis-testing heuristic tells us that the value of a negative test is its ability to rule out a disease. At times, however, we can also use negative tests to point us in the right direction to help us rule in a disease. The problem with using positive tests to rule in disease and negative tests exclusively to rule out disease may not seem obvious, but we may be able to appreciate the bias against the use of negative data if we change George Williams' history a bit.

What if George Williams had been 60 years old and had pain in the pit of his stomach that came and went with a less clear relationship to food? Now pancreatic cancer might have been higher on the differential list. What if we ordered an upper GI for 60-year-old George Williams and it was negative? The negative test would help rule out duodenal ulcer, gastric ulcer, and stomach cancer, but, in addition, we know that an upper GI is usually negative with pancreatic cancer. Thus, this negative data can and should be used for more than ruling out; it should be used to increase the emphasis on ruling in pancreatic cancer. Negative tests do more than rule out a disease; they can raise the probability of other diseases.

## LIMITATIONS OF THE RANGE OF NORMAL

The hypothesis-testing rule-of-thumb assumes that a test is either negative or positive. For many tests such as creatinine, cholesterol, blood pressure, and hematocrit, the results often are not clear-cut positives and negatives. There are many shades of gray. We try to deal with this uncertainty by creating a range of normal. The central 95 percent of values among those believed to be disease free is often used to define a range of normal.* At times the range of normal is set at a level that produces more results outside the range of normal.

The range of normal is developed by selecting a reference group consisting of individuals without known disease. Those individuals may be chosen mainly for convenience, frequently being laboratory personnel or medical students. The test's results for these individuals are then plotted and the central 95 percent is used as the range of normal. Therefore, by definition five percent of the results obtained from these individuals are outside the range of normal.

The range of normal serves as a means of defining, somewhat arbitrarily, which test levels are positive and which are negative. Use of the range of normal to provide positive and negative values for a test leads to a series of potential problems.

*The average value plus or minus two standard deviations is the usual technical definition of the range of normal.

1. Values outside normal limits may not indicate disease since five percent or more of those in the reference group, by definition, have test values outside normal limits. When ordering large numbers of tests, using automated testing, it is an everyday problem to find values outside the range of normal on at least one test—even in the absence of disease. In fact, if 20 tests are performed, one would expect an average of one test result to be outside normal limits even if no disease is present.

2. The range of normal refers to the test values for a specific reference group. Individuals we treat in practice may be different from the reference group used by the laboratory to develop the range of normal. The adult range of alkaline phosphatase is not applicable to children. Granulocyte count for whites doesn't represent the range of normal for blacks. The creatinine of young males is far too high for older women. The hematocrit of women doesn't apply to pregnancy. Yet the laboratory may not inform the clinician of these important facts. If we don't recognize that the usual laboratory range of normal doesn't apply to our specific patient, substantial mistakes can occur when we declare test results positive or negative.

3. Tests within the range of normal merely compare an individual's levels with those of a reference group. They do not say what the individual's value should be. For many tests there is a broad range of normal. The range of serum creatinine is 0.7 to 1.4 mg/ml, the range of normal serum uric acid is 2.5 to 8 mg/ml, the range of hematocrits for males is 42 to 52 percent. Substantial loss of renal function or blood loss may occur as an individual moves from one end to the other of the range of normal. These changes often reflect the develop-

ment of disease. Thus, levels within normal limits may be labeled as negative and hide important pathology.

## OVERRELIANCE ON THE WEIGHT OF THE EVIDENCE

Finally, the hypothesis-testing rule-of-thumb provides little guidance when confronted with multiple tests. When two or more tests are positive we naturally conclude that the disease is more likely than if only one is positive. This is known as reliance on the weight of the evidence. We can rely on the weight of the evidence only if each test result provided additional evidence above and beyond the evidence provided by the first test. This is usually the case only when each test measures disease using different biological phenomenon. For instance, in George Williams' case, endoscopy and upper GI x ray are both means of examining the anatomy to assess the possibility of duodenal ulcer. Doing both tests would have added little to the diagnostic workup designed to identify a duodenal ulcer. Similarly, a sonogram and a computed tomography (CT) scan of the abdomen are both tests for identifying pancreatic cancer. Doing both tests simultaneously adds little to use of the CT scan alone. A negative sonogram, in addition to a negative CT scan will add little to the evidence, though it may produce the bias of overreliance on consistent results.

On the other hand, exercise stress testing, which measures the cardiac electrical activity, and thallium stress testing, which measures the distribution of coronary blood flow, are more likely to produce independent information that can be added together to increase the weight of the evidence.

In addition to overreliance on the weight of the evidence, multiple testing may leave us susceptible to information overload, a phenomenon well-known to many busy practicing physicians. The sensory overload caused by too much data leads to the tendency to ignore both important and unimportant data.

The hypothesis testing rule-of-thumb usually serves us well. However, it requires that we first ask "why are we ordering a test?" It then requires that we make our best estimate of the probability of the disease before ordering a test. In addition, disease identification by hypothesis testing can lead to problems if we fail to fully utilize negative test results; fail to recognize the limitations of positive and negative test results as defined by a range of normal; overrely on the weight of the evidence, or become susceptible to information overload.

## Mistaken Reasons for Ordering Tests

Ordering tests has become so easy in medicine that it usually requires just a touch of the pen. Thus today there are a series of justifications for ordering tests that have little to do with ruling in or ruling out disease. They have a lot to do with the clinician's own fears, anxieties, and tolerance of uncertainty. By ordering tests clinicians may feel like they are doing something. The desire to do something may explain four deceptively attractive reasons for test ordering that lead to many medical mistakes. Tests may be ordered because clinicians:

Can't stand to wait
Have a need "to be complete"
Are scared of lawsuit
Don't know when enough is enough

Time in medicine is often on the side of the doctor and the patient. Self-limited diseases are probably the most common entities encountered in primary care. In addition, many diseases require time to express their full clinical manifestations. The urgency of identifying a disease is, therefore, a function of the potential disease and its consequences and the particular patient. For instance, the level of urgency would be lower in a healthy young man with fever of two days' duration and no localized manifestations than in a man who has an artificial heart valve. Fortunately, clinicians intuitively realize that every problem is not urgent and every delay is not disastrous. At times, intentional delay is valuable if it can be used for careful observation. Observation at its best is a way of using time as a diagnostic test, allowing the pain of a possible gallbladder attack to localize, or the course of an acute fever to become clear. Observation is not mere delay; it implies an active search for new signs and symptoms. For observation to be useful, the types of changes to look for and the timing of follow-up must be outlined in advance. In medicine, clues often appear, rather than disappear, with time.

Clinicians and patients too often assume that they must identify a disease regardless of the difficulties or risks involved. In clinical practice, however, it is often both unnecessary and impractical to obtain an exact disease identification in every case. In some situations, the initial therapy is the same regardless of the disease. There is rarely a need to determine on the first visit the exact disease producing upper respiratory symptoms, acute diarrheal disease, or acute back pain. In other circumstances, the danger of making a specific diagnosis may not be worth the risks. The therapeutic benefit of liver or kidney biopsy needs to be carefully weighed against the risks before the procedure is carried out. Admitting that a problem is of unknown cause may at times be better medicine than subjecting the patient to the risks of identifying a disease. In determining whether to pursue a disease, clinicians must consider what will be done if the disease is identified. The probability, consequences, and reversibility of a potential disease should be assessed before patients are subjected to potentially dangerous tests. In other words, before continuing down the road of extensive testing, clinicians need to step back and ask, "How will the test(s) change what I do?"

In the not too distant past, clinical medicine used the motto "to be complete" to justify ordering many marginal tests. "As long as the patient is in the hospital . . ." "You can never be sure the patient doesn't have disease . . ." "If you think of it, order it." These and other similar phrases were, and may still be, used to justify ordering tests that add little to the diagnostic or therapeutic effort, but plenty to the patient's bill. Ordering "to be complete" is no longer an acceptable approach in an era in which clinicians are under increasing pressure to be efficient.

Clinicians often fear that they will look bad in court if they fail to make a diagnosis. This leads to the practice of "defensive medicine" in which clinicians order tests because they are scared of a lawsuit. Tests ordered when a disease is already unlikely can cause more trouble than they are worth. Often the majority of positive tests in this situation are false positives.* In this situation the probability

---

*Imagine a test with 90 percent sensitivity and 85 percent specificity. This test is comparable to many tests used to identify disease. If there is a ten percent probability of disease before performing the test, then the probability of disease after obtaining a positive test (the predictive value of a positive test) can be calculated using the following table:*

*10% Prior Probability*

|  | *Disease (+)* | *Disease (−)* |
|---|---|---|
| *Test (+)* | *90* | *135* |
| *Test (−)* | *10* | *765* |
|  | *100* | *900* |

*The probability of disease after obtaining a positive test =*

$$\frac{90}{90 + 135} = 40\%.$$ *Thus the majority (60%) of the positive tests in this situation are false positive.*

of a false-positive result necessitates further, sometimes dangerous testing, to rule out the disease. Malpractice suits rarely have anything to do with the failure to order tests; they are usually, at least for primary care physicians, about the breakdown of the doctor-patient relationship. There are often better forms of protection from malpractice suit than ordering more tests, as we shall discuss in Chapter 13.

Closely related to the fear of lawsuit, however, is the desire to order tests to provide reassurance. This practice is tempting, but remember that in the situation of low probability of disease, positive test results are usually false positives, unless the test has sensitivity and specificity approaching 100 percent. The electrocardiogram ordered to provide a patient with reassurance may backfire and lead down an unproductive and dangerous path. Alternatively, it may falsely reassure the patient that coronary artery disease is not present. Testing to provide reassurance must be done very selectively since it often makes medicine more difficult. The reassurance of close follow-up is often the best reassurance for the doctor and the patient.

Deciding when enough is enough is one of the most difficult decisions a physician must make. In deciding to stop, physicians need to ask whether further testing is likely to alter what will be done. It is standard practice to treat most cancers only after obtaining biopsy evidence of the specific pathology. Thus, in general, not enough has been done until tissue is obtained, even when evidence points strongly to a diagnosis of cancer and the uncertainty is low. Often, however, initial treatment can be instituted based on a tentative diagnosis, and further diagnostic efforts can await the patient's response. This approach has been called the threshold approach to disease identification. Clinicians set a threshold defining how certain they need to be before tentatively identifying a disease and proceeding with treatment. The threshold will differ for each disease depending on the difficulty of diagnosis and the dangers of treatment.

Thus clinicians must consciously make the decision when enough is enough. Usually the key is to remember that stopping is not a permanent decision; it can and should be continually reevaluated. With multiple opportunities to do more testing, it is often easier to say "enough for now."

Now that we have identified a disease, let us step back and look at what we've found. Physicians usually are asked to identify a disease according to a set of criteria defined by the medical profession. It is not usually a physician's job to ask "what is a disease anyway?" However, in an era of rapid change it is worth thinking about what we mean by a disease, since for many diseases the very definition is changing before our eyes. New technology alters our concepts of mitral valve prolapse and pituitary adenomas. New knowledge of genetics forces us to reclassify diseases, including many cancers, and to subdivide others, such as diabetes mellitus. New knowledge of the natural history of diseases alters the criteria for identifying AIDS and Lyme disease. To understand how the definition of a disease can change, we need to understand how diseases are defined. Diseases have usually been defined using three different types of approaches.

1. Deviation from socially acceptable function: Social-cultural approach
2. Deviations from usual function: The statistical approach
3. Deviations from proper function: The functional approach

Defining disease by social functioning is often an initial way to classify disease, especially when that is all we have to go on. Defining disease by socially acceptable functioning has in recent times been used to classify drug abuse, child abuse, and alcohol abuse as diseases. Despite the need for this approach, its dangers should be recognized. Social values in the nineteenth century, for instance, classified masturbation as a disease. Likewise, homosexuality was classified as a disease until recent years.

Thus a condition may be defined as disease or nondisease depending on the social values of a society. As these ideas or values change, disease may be classified as nondisease and vice versa.

Often, diseases are defined not by how society thinks people should function but by how they have been found to usually function. Disease may be defined as deviations from usual function using a statistical approach.

The statistical approach may be used to define a subgroup of individuals as different. This difference may be used at least temporarily to define a disease. Levels of blood sugar and hematocrit have been used to define diabetes mellitus and anemia before these numbers could be translated into a deviation from proper functioning. The dangers of using statistical definitions of disease are that the levels may be set too high or too low. When statistical concepts of disease are used it is possible to dismiss clinical manifestations, such as smokers cough, as common and innocent symptoms. In recent years the definition of high blood pressure and high cholesterol have had to be altered in recognition that more than five percent of the population is at risk of vascular disease from elevation of blood pressure and cholesterol. The statistical concept of disease thus assumes that the usual level among individuals without apparent problems is the desirable level. This statistical concept is reflected in the use of the range of normal.

The dangers of the statistical definition of disease

also go the other way. As our technology becomes more sophisticated we find more individuals with deviations such as cerebral atropy, renal masses, and mitral valve prolapse. Do these individuals have a disease? Not necessarily. Before these individuals have been extensively studied, it is tempting to classify them as having disease. However, it is important to remember that there may be severe social consequences of labelling cerebral atropy a disease. The cost of working up nonprogressive renal masses may be very high. The dangers of antibiotic prophylaxis for all patients with mitral valve prolapse can be substantial. Thus, like the social-cultural definition of a disease, the statistical approach is less than ideal.

Deviation from proper functioning as identified by signs or symptoms on clinical evaluation has been the most common way we define disease. Increasingly, however, we are attempting to identify diseases before there are any apparent clinical deviation from proper functioning. To achieve this goal we must understand enough about the outcome of disease processes and human functioning to know what is proper. Increasingly disease is defined by current test values that are believed to predict future deviations from proper functioning in the absence of intervention. Elevated prolactin or thyroid stimulating hormones may be considered disease even in the absence of signs or symptoms.

Diseases are being subdivided into categories that over time may be considered separate diseases, especially if their prognosis and treatment diverge. This evolution can be seen in the case of diabetes mellitus. Diabetes mellitus was for many years regarded as a single disease ch. ᵃacterized by elevations in blood sugar; a statistical definition of disease. The advent of hemoglobin AIC has allowed us to take a more functional approach to the definition of the disease well before there is evidence of functional problems at the clinical level. In addition, the disease has been divided into Type I insulin dependent, Type II noninsulin dependent, and most recently Type III associated with at least 60 genetic syndromes. Increasingly these categories are being subdivided based on a more precise understanding of function. Function may be disturbed, for example, by abnormalities of insulin production, genetically determined structural abnormalities of the insulin molecule, or abnormalities at the receptor level. Each of these refinements help to pinpoint our definition of the disease and help the definition of disease serve as the basis for prognosis and treatment. What is clear to the clinician is that the definition of diabetes mellitus is constantly changing. Having identified a disease, and explored what we mean by a disease, let us turn to the last step in the process, that of providing an explanation.

# 6

# *Explanation:*
## *From Cause to Clinical Manifestations*

Increasingly, high-tech medicine is making disease identification easier. Having identified a disease, clinicians may be satisfied that the job is done. However, disease identification is not the same as diagnosis. A diagnosis usually requires more than the identification of a disease. In some conditions, such as pregnancy, a diagnosis does not imply a disease at all if we regard a disease as a deviation from proper functioning. A diagnosis outlines what is known about the processes leading to the patient's symptoms. A diagnosis helps us to understand what is going on in a specific clinical situation, how and why it has occurred, and what it means for the future. Ideally, a diagnosis provides a basis for evaluating potential therapies. The process of arriving at a diagnosis is really the process of attempting to explain what is occurring. This process relies heavily on our basic scientific understanding of disease mechanisms. As Kassirer writes:

> . . . (physiologic) reasoning remains a fundamental underpinning of diagnostic reasoning, and, when applicable, it enhances the diagnostic process with the richness of its explanatory power.[12]

Thus a full diagnosis is an explanation that may be thought of as requiring three components:

Clinical manifestations
Disease
Cause

We can use the acronym CDC to remember these components. This CDC approach can be a very useful way of putting together what we know, and forcing us to direct our attention to the relationship between the clinical manifestations of the disease and the underlying cause.

These distinctions between causes, disease, and clinical manifestation are given labels in the field of genetics. The gene abnormality of **genotype** is regarded as the cause of the disease itself. The **phenotype** is the disease, the genetic product that can be measured. The **genetic expressivity** indicates the clinical manifestations of the disease. The same genetic product may result in a spectrum from asymptomatic to severe clinical manifestations.

Thus, completing the diagnostic process requires us to identify an explanation that provides the linkages among:

Cause ------------>   Disease ------------>   Clinical
                                             manifestation

To complete a diagnosis once a disease has been identified we must ask:

1. Is the identified disease(s) the explanation of the patient's clinical manifestations?
2. Is there a known cause that is the explanation of the patient's disease(s)?

Cause is a difficult concept that may mean different things to different people. The concept of cause is confusing because diseases may have more than one cause, and the presence of a cause does not ensure the development of a disease. A clinically useful concept of cause is known as contributory cause. Establishing contributory cause requires demonstrating that:

The cause and the disease are associated; they occur together more frequently than expected by chance alone
The cause precedes the disease in time
Altering the cause alters the effect

The first criterion is usually established not at the individual level, but based on studies of groups of individuals. Thus, in George Williams' case, we draw on medical knowledge to obtain the association between alcohol and duodenal ulcer. In assessing whether the cause preceded the effect, we evaluate not only whether George Williams drank prior to developing a duodenal ulcer, but whether the quantity and timing was consistent. One night of heavy drinking, for instance, would not be likely to produce a duodenal ulcer. A pattern of chronic alcohol use with increased use on weekends, however, is consistent with the development of a duodenal ulcer. Establishing the third criterion—altering the cause alters the effect—is often the most difficult part of establishing contributory cause. Often it can only be presumed in retrospect, perhaps after George Williams stops drinking and the ulcer does not recur. Often cause must continue to be presumed based on our best guesses. We cannot be certain that alcohol was the cause of George Williams' ulcer. There may be other causes as well. Even in what seems like straightforward disease, it is important to recognize that the explanation may not be so simple. Duodenal ulcers may be part of hyperparathyroidism, for instance, which itself can be part of multiple endocrine neoplasia syndromes. Alternatively, there must always be a first ulcer in a disease characterized by recurrent duodenal ulcers such as the Zollinger-Ellison syndrome. Experienced clinicians do not immediately order a gastrin level even after recognizing the possibility of Zollinger-Ellison syndrome. However, if the ulcer fails to heal or recurs their minds remain open to this possible explanation.

Now that we have distinguished cause from disease and disease from clinical manifestations, let us take a look at a series of diagnostic descriptions using this CDC approach to diagnosis.

Example 1:
**C:** Cough and shortness of breath
**D:** Emphysema
**C:** Cigarette smoking–50 pack-years

The first example provides an explanation for the cough and shortness of breath as due to a disease. Emphysema implies a specific, pathologic pattern with a corresponding set of consistent clinical finding, pulmonary functions, and x ray results. The emphysema itself is explained by the preceding 50 pack-years of cigarette smoking.

Example 2:
**C:** Exertional chest pains: unstable

**D:** 90 percent obstruction of the left main coronary artery

**C:** Hypertension and hyperlipidemia

In the second example we are declaring that the 90 percent obstruction of the left main coronary artery is the explanation of the exertional chest pain. It also implies that the patient's hypertension and hyperlipidemia are both contributory causes of the disease.

The CDC approach requires us to distinguish between a disease and a cause. Here again we need to ask what is a disease. For instance, hyperlipidemia is increasingly being regarded as a disease in terms of deviations from proper functioning. Thus, the distinction between a cause and a disease can at times be artificial, and it may depend on the question being asked.

The CDC approach to disease diagnosis forces us to integrate our knowledge from a variety of medical disciplines. It requires us to correlate the anatomy, physiology, biochemistry, and epidemiology with the clinical disease manifestations to produce an adequate and coherent explanation.

In many clinical situatons, the CDC format will not be able to be filled in as completely as these previous examples suggest. At times there may be nothing to say in one of the categories.

Example 3:
**C:** Asymptomatic
**D:** Increased serum uric acid
**C:** Overproduction of uric acid

In this example there are no clinical manifestations of the increased serum level of uric acid. The explicit acknowledgement of an absence of clinical manifestations helps us recognize the difference between the presence of a disease and the presence of current clinical manifestations. If a painful joint with uric acid crystals were present, then we could have labelled the clinical manifestations as gout. Without symptoms we must be careful to limit ourselves to designation of a disease defined by elevated serum uric acid.

The need to link a disease with the clinical manifestations and to link it with an underlying cause has long been recognized by practicing physicians and accomplished with the assistance of the rule-of-thumb known as the *principle of parsimony*. Most of the time the principle of parsimony helps us by suggesting a single diagnosis linking a cause, disease, and clinical manifestations. The physician then can put together a coherent and adequate explanation of the patient's diagnosis diagrammed as follows:

| Explanation<br>of disease | Explanation of Clinical<br>manifestations | |
|---|---|---|
| Cause ------------> | Disease ------------> | Clinical<br>manifestations |

Use of the principle of parsimony is usually accomplished by clinicians themselves. When the pieces don't all fit easily together, however, we must step back and look for new ways to put them together. Sometimes patients' ideas may be critical to putting the pieces together. Often it is helpful to elicit a patient's ideas by asking, "How do you fit this all together?" or "What do you think is going on here?" The clinician may be greatly assisted by the patient who answers, "Could my wife's death explain all this?" or, "Could these medications be causing all my problems?" At other times these questions may bring out realistic or unrealistic fears of sexually transmitted disease or cancer.

Exclusive reliance on the principle of parsimony to link disease with symptoms and cause with disease is prone to a series of potential problems.

Failure to systematically determine whether a disease is actually the explanation of the patient's symptoms

Failure to recognize that multiple disease may exist in the same individual, and that not all diseases produce clinical manifestations

Failure to acknowledge the uncertainty that remains

## DETERMINING WHETHER A DISEASE IS THE EXPLANATION OF THE SYMPTOMS

How do clinicians know when a disease is actually the explanation of a patient's symptoms? In theory we use the same three criteria that we used to establish that a cause explains a disease. Here the disease must be associated with the clinical manifestations, the disease precedes the clinical manifestations, and altering the disease alters the clinical manifestations. Medical literature tells us if specific clinical manifestations may be part of the disease. Further, the presence of the disease must precede the development of the clinical manifestations. Usually these first two criteria are relatively easy to establish. However, to definitively establish that the disease is actually the explanation of the patient's clinical manifestations requires more than a compatible disease. Clinicians need to determine whether altering the disease alters the symptoms.

Unfortunately, establishing that altering the disease alters the clinical manifestations is not always so easy or safe to accomplish. For instance, to establish that a drug allergy is present, a typical rash that is thought to be a side effect of a particular drug may be identified. Removal of the drug, with disappearance of the rash, helps confirm drug allergy as the explanation of the rash. Establishing definitively that the drug is the explanation of the rash, however, would require blind readministration of the drug with reappearance of the rash. While this may be an intellectually satisfying means of explaining the symptoms, it can be a dangerous method. Thus, often we must live with the uncertainty and settle for a less than definite answer.

Despite the difficulties, in many instances, it is possible to obtain evidence that altering the disease alters the symptoms. This can be done by using a variety of techniques, including physical examination maneuvers, formal testing procedures, therapeutic trials, and careful observation.

Physical examination procedures are the most commonly used techniques for explaining the clinical manifestations. For instance, reproduction of a patient's symptoms by rapid breathing (known as hyperventilation) and disappearance of the symptoms by slow rebreathing into a paper bag help confirm that hyperventilation is the explanation of a patient's symptoms.

High-tech medicine has done more to assist in disease identification than in establishing explanation of symptoms. However, emphasis has recently been placed on what we will call explanation testing that alters the anatomy or physiology and observes the effects on symptoms. Drugs may be carefully administered to induce spasm of the esophagus, bronchial airways, or spasm of the coronary arteries to determine whether the patient's symptoms are reproduced. While these tests may be informative they may also carry substantial risk.

At times the best means of establishing an explanation of clinical manifestations is to treat the disease and see the effect. This method of explaining symptoms is called a therapeutic trial. Therapeutic trials must be carefully performed with active participation by the patient. To be useful in explaining symptoms, patients must know what to watch for as well as when and what to report back to the clinician.

At times it is more judicious to rely on careful observation of the patient's course to determine whether the disease is the explanation of the patient's symptoms. Time is often the most useful of diagnostic tests. The spontaneous resolution of diarrhea, abdominal pain, upper respiratory symptoms, or back pain may provide valuable retrospective information. It allows the clinician to explain the symptoms, or at least be reassured by resolution of the symptoms, that no progressive problem is occurring. Observation, however, like a therapeutic trial, requires the doctor, and often the patient, to know what to look for and how and when to look for it. For instance, a clinician may treat acute nausea and vomiting occurring in several family members as acute gastroenteritis or stomach flu, advising clear liquids and observation. To fully accomplish observation, the patient needs to be prepared to look for the symptoms of dehydration, such as lightheadedness, and for signs of bleeding, such as coffee ground vomiting or black tarry stools. Finally, the patient should be told to expect rapid resolution of the vomiting within 12 to 24 hours, and if symptoms continue to obtain a follow-up evaluation.

As we have seen, the explanation of the clinical manifestation is separate and distinct from the question of the presence of a disease. Determining that the clinical symptoms can be explained by the disease may be established using physical examination, explanation testing, therapeutic trials, and careful observation to determine whether altering the disease alters the symptoms, or altering the cause alters the disease.

## MULTIPLE DISEASES AND NO CLINICAL MANIFESTATION OF A DISEASE

The principle of parsimony does not adequately account for the increasingly frequent occurrence of multiple diseases in the same individual. The existence of multiple diseases in a single individual is becoming an increasingly common clinical phenomenon. More individuals are living to an older age, and therapeutic interventions keep individuals alive while leaving them susceptible to additional diseases.

Cause -------> Disease

Clinical Manifestations

Cause -------> Disease

If not used carefully, the principle of parsimony can imply that if a disease could be producing a patient's symptom, it is producing these symptoms. For instance, a physician may uncover diverticulum or gallstones in an evaluation of abdominal pain, but these diseases may have little or no relationship to a patient's symptoms. A second unrecognized disease may be producing the clinical manifestation.

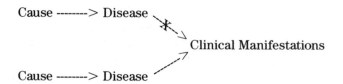

Cause -------> Disease

Clinical Manifestations

Cause -------> Disease

In addition, the principle of parsimony does not deal with the rapidly accumulating number of conditions that can be detected at an early stage when clinical manifestations are absent. It has long been recognized that patients may be asymptomatic despite the presence of such potentially progressive diseases as tuberculosis, syphilis, coronary artery disease, and cirrhosis. In addition, medicine's rapidly expanding technology has increasingly enabled the identification of diseases such as hyperparathyroidism and hyperprolactinoma at a stage where they do not produce, and may never produce, symptoms or other consequences.

Cause ------------> Disease ------X------> No Clinical
                                          Manifesta-
                                          tions

## ACKNOWLEDGING THE UNCERTAINTY THAT REMAINS

Medicine is recognizing that if we look hard enough and closely enough most people have evidence of disease. Some diseases progress, others are cured "spontaneously," and still other coexist with the individual during many years of active life. Most of us will die **of** a disease, but will also die **with** many other diseases.

Social disability can result from identification of a condition even when it is not associated with clinical manifestations. Children may be disabled by a functional heart murmur. Mild hypertension may result in increased work disability when none would be expected medically. The "medicalization" of conditions like mitral valve prolapse may turn a generally benign condition, one that may be a normal variant, into a disease with substantial social and medical consequences.

Resisting the tendency to identify a disease may be difficult, but tolerating the subsequent uncertainty is often better than making a diagnosis based on insufficient data. A possible pulmonary emboli, or a possible duodenal ulcer, becomes a definite emboli or ulcer when remembered by the patient or evaluated by the next physician. Symptoms can be idenfied as problems on a problem list while avoiding the tendency to identify a disease. A problem list might include chronic abdominal pain of unknown etiology or chest pain without evidence of progressive disease. These positive assertions of the existence of uncertainty alert the next clinician not to be overconfident.

Having determined the presence of one or more diseases, and having assessed whether the disease or diseases explain the patient's symptoms, it should be possible to step back a minute and put together a complete diagnosis.

Remember, a diagnosis aims to explain the patient's symptoms by linking together three basic entities:

1. A patient's clinical manifestations—the symptoms, signs, and laboratory results.
2. One or more diseases ideally defined as deviation from proper functioning, which are the explanations of a patient's clinical manifestation.
3. The cause(s) or the entity that explains the occurrence of disease.

Use of the CDC approach helps us define what we know and what we don't know. Often there will be blanks because we just don't know the cause or are not sure about the connections.

At other times the inability to fill in the CDC of a diagnosis may be due to the medical community's lack of understanding of underlying causes. For instance, in example 4 a headache that has the characteristic of a classic migraine would be depicted in the CDC classification as follows:

Example 4:
**C:** Unilateral throbbing headache with preceding visual symptoms
**D:** Classic migraine
**C:** Unknown

Again, this approach outlines our understanding

of the clinical manifestations and the disease. In addition, it requires us to acknowledge our lack of understanding of the basic cause of migraine headaches. While we hope that increased clinical skills and increased basic scientific knowledge will allow us to more completely fill in the CDCs, we also need to learn the art and science of living with the uncertainty that lies at the heart of medical decision making.

Acknowledging uncertainty helps us keep our minds open to new data and new approaches since medical understanding is in a constant state of evolution. Even in a straightforward situation like George Williams—with epigastric pain, duodenal ulcer, and alcohol abuse—there may actually have been another previously unappreciated cause of his problem. Recent evidence suggests that helicobacter pylori infection may produce a chronic, antral gastritis, predisposing these patients by an unknown mechanism to duodenal ulcer.

Clinicians learn by experience as well as training to rapidly proceed through the five steps of the SHADE approach—from symptoms, to hunch, to alternatives, to disease, to explanation. The process often becomes second nature, so that we have difficulty describing what we are doing. Like an experienced baseball pitcher, we have difficulty describing how we throw our pitches. Much of what has been learned about the process of diagnosis comes from studies that observed experienced physicians evaluating patient problems. The physicians were asked to stop multiple times during the evaluation to convey what they were thinking. It was at first a bit surprising to many that did not follow the time-honored method taught in medical school. The physicians did not first collect all the data, then step back and evaluate it. Rather, they engaged in an active process of information gathering and active thinking about the data along the way.

After an initial brief period of letting patients set

the stage, these physicians formed initial hunches or hypotheses, and their remaining questioning was largely based on the hypothesis. Questioning was said to be hypotheses driven. This starting and stopping method helped us recognize that diagnosis does not move smoothly from step 1 to step 5. Clinicians recycle along the way. Before making a diagnosis, a clinician may recycle through the five steps, gathering additional data, confirming the quality of his or her data, and seeing how it all fits together. This recycling has been called an iterative process. The diagnostic process is therefore an active, hypothesis driven, iterative process. Thus the diagnostic process is in constant motion. However, an effort to sort out what occurs during each of the five steps of the diagnostic process can be helpful. Equipped with an understanding of these steps, students and even experienced physicians can sit back and learn from what we do everyday.

## REFERENCES

1. Tversky A, Kahneman D. Judgement under uncertainty. *Heuristics and Biases Science.* 185:1124–31, 1974.

2. Burack RC, Carpenter RR. The predictive value of the presenting complaint. *J Fam Pract* 16(4):749–54, 1983.

3. Barsky AJ. Hidden reasons some patients visit doctors. *Ann Intern Med* 94:492–8, 1981.

4. Young M. Society for General Internal Medicine Newsletter. Vol. 10(4) Sept-Oct, 1987. P. 7.

5. Enelow AJ, Swisher SN. *Interviewing and Patient Care.* New York; Oxford University Press, 1986.

6. Albert DA, Munson, R, Resnik, MD. *Reasoning in Medicine.* Baltimore: The Johns Hopkins University Press, 1988. P. 201.

7. Tumulty PA. The Effective Clinician: His Methods and Approach to Diagnosis and Care. Philadelphia: Saunders, 1973.

8. Schwartz S, Griffin T. *Medical Thinking: The Psychology of Medical Judgment and Decision Making.* New York: Springer-Verlag, 1986. P. 36–38.

9. Desmond M. *Manwatching: A Field Guide to Human Behavior.* New York: Harry H. Abrahm, 1977.

10. Arkes HN. Impediments to accurate judgment and possible ways to minimize the impact. *J Consult Clin Psychol* 49(3):323–333, 1980.

11. Hardison JE. To be complete. *N Engl J Med.* 300:193–4, 1979.

12. Kassirer JP. Diagnostic reasoning. *Ann Intern Med* 110:896, 1988.

# II

# Bothering with the PESTER Process

# 7

# *Prediction*

Making a correct diagnosis is too often regarded as the ultimate intellectual challenge in medicine. Once a diagnosis has been made and the patient is correctly labelled, physicians too often consider the challenge of medical care complete. With diagnosis a sophisticated intellectual process is often required to reach a conclusion. With therapy it is tempting to merely look up the official recommendations of experts, using a cookbook approach.

The selection and implementation of therapy, however, is a far more complicated and dynamic process than is apparent from the attention it has traditionally received in medical schools. Selecting the right treatment for the right patient and maximizing the benefits of treatment require a systematic approach to what needs to be done, what can go wrong, and how to minimize mistakes.

Clinicians who are successful in the therapeutic process usually take the time and bother to follow a logical step-by-step process. These steps can be combined into the mnemonic PESTER.

The PESTER process stands for:

Prediction: Predicting future disease and the future course of current disease in the absence of treatment.

Effectiveness: Assessing the effectiveness and cost effectiveness of potential therapies for the individual patient and groups of patients.

Safety: Assessing the safety of potential therapies for the individual patient.

Therapeutic Decision: Developing therapeutic recommendations and engaging the patient in informed consent.

Execution: Implementing the therapy to maximize its benefits and minimize its risks.

Reflection: Monitoring the outcome of therapy and reassessing the treatment based on any less than expected results.

Let us take a look at why it is worth the time and effort to bother with the PESTER process. We will look at what is required for each step in the process and what needs to be done to prevent problems along the way.

The goal of clinical prediction is to make our best estimates of an individual's clinical course or natural history in the absence of treatment. This prediction then can be used to determine how the outcome may be altered by interventions.

Feinstein has emphasized the key role that prediction plays in clinical medicine saying, "In the basic science of patient care, prediction is as important for managerial decisions as explanation has become for decisions about pathogenesis and diagnosis of disease[1]." The ability to predict the course of disease was the focus of much of medical education in the early twentieth century. Long before physicians had the sophisticated technologies to diagnose many diseases or the therapeutic advances to alter the course of disease, physicians were often able to predict the immediate course of disease. As Lewis Thomas has written in *The Youngest Science*, "In the early twentieth century, the art of prediction needed education and was the sole contribution of the medical school; good medical schools produced doctors who knew enough of the details of the natural history of disease to be able to make reliable prognosis[2]."

This century has brought about tremendous advances in diagnosis and therapy. As physicians' attentions have been turned to diagnosis and therapy, much less attention has been directed to clinical prediction.

There are really two types of prediction, risk analysis and prognosis. Risk analysis looks at the probability of developing a disease. In contrast, we will use the word prognosis to mean the type of prediction that we make once a disease is present. It predicts the probability of developing complications of a disease. Prognosis is the link between diagnosis and therapy. These two concepts can be integrated into our CDC of a diagnosis:

Cause ------------> Disease ------------> Clinical
                                            manifestations
    Risk Analysis        Prognosis

## RISK ANALYSIS

Recognition that risk analysis is really a separate form of prediction helps us avoid the common medical mindset that mistakenly focuses only on avoiding complications of current disease, rather than aiming to prevent the occurrence of disease in the first place. Failure to provide prevention is one of the most common errors in clinical medicine. In order to focus our preventive efforts on those most likely to benefit, it is important to define patient characteristics known as risk factors that increase the probability of disease. Data from groups of individuals allow us to identify risk factors. These risk factors may include characteristics such as hypertension or cigarette smoking, which may be causes of disease and can be changed, or factors such as age and sex that cannot be changed. Having recognized the existence of a potentially reversible risk factor, we can often use that information to intervene early to identify and treat disease. This strategy has worked well for hypertension, for instance, and is now being aggressively pursued for hyperlipidemia. Risk factors such as age and sex may be used to identify patients for screening programs such as breast cancer screening in which early detection and early treatment are the goals.

It is important to recognize, however, that early intervention will not always be successful. Problems occur with early intervention:

When lead-time bias is the reason for the apparent success of early intervention
When length bias is the reason for the apparent success of early intervention

## Lead-time Bias

Early intervention assumes there is successful therapy that will be more useful if used at an earlier stage in the disease process. At times this is not the case. For instance, early identification of lung cancer among smokers using routine chest x rays and cytology has not been shown to improve the outcome of the disease. The time between disease identification and death, however, is increased, producing what is called a lead-time bias. Increased lead time is what early intervention is all about. However, there must be treatment available that can be more successfully applied during the extra time provided. If this is not the case then all that is gained is an earlier recognition of a bad outcome.

Intervention to alter risk factors before the appearance of disease may still be too late to head off the occurrence of the disease. For instance, five years after menopause the benefits of replacement estrogen for prevention of osteoporosis are minimal. Thus while early intervention to increase lead time is often an excellent strategy, at times it may not work because the treatment is not successful or even early treatment is too late.

## Length Bias

Early intervention may appear to work because screening may detect large numbers of cases of slowly progressive disease. Even if not detected, many of these would never become clinically apparent. Aggressive screening for certain cancers, such as prostate and thyroid, would undoubtedly increase the number of cancers detected and the number "cured." It is not so clear that these cancers, if left undetected, would endanger the patient. Thus, in these situations it is not clear that aggressive screening would reduce the development of clinical disease. As our diagnostic tools improve we have more and more opportunities to identify risk factors and to detect early disease. However, unless we are alert to the natural history of disease and the existence of many indolent, nonprogressive, well-controlled diseases, we may advocate early intervention even when it is not necessary.

When identifying risk factors and measuring their impact, it is important to recognize two important sources of misinterpretation and potential error:

The impact of a risk factor requires us to consider the magnitude of the risk and not just the relative risk.

The existence of multiple risk factors may dramatically increase the risk. At times the risk may be greatly reduced by reduction or elimination of only one risk factor.

## Relative Risk

The relative risk is a measure of the probability of developing a disease if the risk factor is present, divided by the probability of developing the disease if the risk factor is absent. If the presence of a risk factor such as birth control pills increases the risk of thrombophlebitis tenfold, compared to the probability in the absence of birth control pills, use of birth control pills is said to carry a relative risk of 10. We may speak in terms of relative risk even when there is no evidence that the risk factor is a cause of the disease. However, when a contributory cause of thrombophlebitis such as birth control pills is under consideration, the relative risk is a useful measure for individual decision making. A relative risk of 10 then says to the individual woman: If you are like the average woman, you will have ten times the probability of developing thrombophelbitis if you are taking the pill compared to your probability of thrombophlebitis if you are not taking the pill.

This relative risk, however, may mean very different things for different patients. A relative risk of 10 may mean that the risk increases from 1 per 1,000,000 to 10 per 1,000,000 or it may mean an increase from 1 per 100 to 10 per 100. Thus, for instance, when advising a patient on the risk of developing complications from birth control pills, the same tenfold increase in risk may have very different implications for a 35-year-old woman with hypertension and a history of thrombophlebitis compared to a 20-year-old woman with a negative past history.

## Multiple Risk Factors

When a patient has two or more risk factors for a disease we need to appreciate how they might interact. The same risk factor such as cigarette smoking may interact very differently in different situations. The effects of some risk factors are multiplicative, that is, the risk from one is multiplied by the risk from the other. For instance, this is the case for cigarette smoking and asbestos exposure as risk factors for lung cancer. If the relative risk of prolonged asbestos exposure is 5, and the relative risk of prolonged cigarette exposure is 10, then the relative risk when both exposures occur together is 50. When risk factors are multiplicative, elimination of either one can have an enormous impact on the risk of disease.

With mesothelioma as opposed to lung cancer, however, the addition of cigarette smoking to asbestos exposure does not increase the risk over exposure to asbestos alone. At other times the risk factors may be additive. The relative risks of cigarette smoking, hypertension, and high cholesterol add one on top of the other to increase the relative risk of coronary artery disease. Thus failure to pay attention to how risk factors interact can lead to problems interpreting risk.

## PROGNOSIS

Once a disease is present we would like to be able to formulate a prognosis. The aim of prognosis is to predict the future course of the disease for the individual patient. As with risk analysis we use data from groups of individuals. With prognosis, however, we also include information we have available about the individual themself. Our ability to assess prognosis for the individual, however, is often very limited, especially when it comes to predicting the long-term consequences for a particular disease in a particular patient. Even when predicting which patients with incurable cancers will live six months,

Forster and Lynn have shown that internists, oncologists, and social workers do equally poorly, achieving results that are little better than could be expected by chance alone[3]. Thus, often our interest in prognosis must focus on the immediate future, on what we will call the immediate clinical prognosis.

Studies of groups of individuals with well-defined diseases have helped us to identify objectively measured prognostic factors that help us predict the outcome of a disease, just as risk factors help predict the development of a disease. These prognostic factors have been used to divide patients into stages or classes of disease such as the stages of cancer or classes of heart disease. Groups of individuals classified according to these stages or classes can then be studied to determine how therapeutic interventions compare with the results obtained when we merely observe the natural history of the disease.

Within any group of individuals who share a common group prognosis, however, there will be some who do better than others. Individual prognosis depends on a wide variety of factors, many of which we are only beginning to understand. Predictions about individuals are particularly difficult clinical tasks. The clinical information necessary for estimating an individual's prognosis may not always be expressed in easily measurable or quantifiable terms; for instance; the patient's nutritional status, degree of disability, family support system, or will to live all contribute to his or her prognosis.

One means of integrating the individual's situation with the group prognosis is to assess the direction an individual is going and the speed with which he or she is moving there. To accomplish this we must specifically address the issues of severity and urgency of the patient's disease. Let us take a more in-depth look at what is necessary to accurately assess the severity and urgency of a patient's problem, and look at some common mistakes in formulating an immediate clinical prognosis.

## SERIOUSNESS

At times the seriousness of a disease is readily apparent to physicians. A blood pressure of 200/140 and a blood pressure of 145/95 are both labeled hypertension; clinicians, however, usually instinctively recognize the differences in severity. The assessment of seriousness is not always so straightforward as reading the numbers. Errors in assessing the seriousness of a disease may occur when we are misled by:

The intensity of symptoms
The direction of the numbers
Overreliance on the laboratory findings

The intensity of symptoms can be misleading since it is often based on a patient's propensity to express or suppress symptoms. Patients experiencing the same condition will express quite different degrees of pain. Awareness of cultural differences in patterns of expressing pain can help us interpret a patient's response. Often asking patients how this pain compares to others they have experienced, such as in childbirth or after surgery, will serve as a better judge of the intensity of the pain. Some of the most medically important conditions may not be associated with intense pain. On the other hand, less life-threatening conditions such as uncomplicated kidney stones are among the most painful of conditions, yet initial treatment can often be limited to relief of pain. Disease complications may actually be heralded by relief of pain with persistence of pathology. A kidney stone that continues to obstruct the ureter after the pain subsides indicates a far more serious disease. In some situations relief of pain may be a bad prognostic sign. For instance, temporary relief of pain after acute peptic ulcer perforation usually occurs prior to the onset of life-threatening peritonitis.

Seriousness should not be assessed exclusively by looking at the laboratory values and determining how far outside the range of normal they are, or even by asking whether they are moving toward the range of normal. Improvement in the numbers may actually be a bad prognostic sign. In overwhelming hepatic necrosis, for instance, the liver enzymes actually fall as the viable hepatocytes are exhausted. The clinical status then becomes a better indicator of the seriousness of the disease.

When the laboratory result does not correlate with what we can tell from examining and talking with the patient, the laboratory results may be misleading. For instance, in pericardial tamponade due to acute trauma, infections, or spontaneous bleeding, the echocardiogram may reveal only a small amount of pericardial fluid. The diagnosis and emergency treatment of tamponade thus relies on the clinical assessment of severity.

Mild symptoms may be the clinical manifestations of serious disease. False reassurance can occur when the extent of disease appears to be minimal or transient. The minimal and transient nature of the shortness of breath due to a small pulmonary embolus, or the brief episode of weakness due to a transient ischemic attack, may falsely reassure the patient and the physician.

## URGENCY

Urgency and seriousness are often closely linked. However, they are separate concepts that require a separate assessment. Seriousness implies that morbidity or mortality is likely. Urgency implies that consequences are imminent. The assessment of urgency requires the physician to ask which manifestations of the disease are the most immediately life threatening. The assessment of urgency is so critical that a consideration of urgency often appropriately precedes a full diagnosis. Errors in assessment of urgency are potentially life threatening since they lead physicians to misplaced priorities. Among the types of errors in assessing urgency are:

Placing diagnosis ahead of urgent treatment
Placing relief of symptoms ahead of urgent evaluation and treatment
The tendency to equate the need for urgent therapy with the degree of laboratory abnormalities

Grave consequences can result from placing diagnosis ahead of urgent treatment. It is obvious to most physicians that a patient with copious hematemesis may require blood replacement prior to definitive diagnosis. It may be less obvious that a patient with head trauma requires immediate evaluation and treatment of intercranial pressure prior to a thorough diagnostic assessment. Patients presenting unconscious should usually be given IV glucose and narcotic antagonists even when these conditions are unlikely. Many manifestations of disease are initially treated similarly, regardless of the exact etiology. Acute intestinal obstruction requires decompression while the exact cause is being pursued. Severe hyperkalemia needs rapid reduction regardless of the cause. Withholding treatment until the diagnosis is clear can be a life-threatening error in the assessment of urgency. Patients do not die of the disease itself, rather they die of physiologic disruptions or secondary infection. Efforts to formulate an immediate clinical prognosis and implement therapy based on that prognosis often have more to do

with the outcome in critically ill patients than
initially making the right diagnosis.

Recognizing the urgency of treatment, however, is
different from urgently treating the painful or aggra-
vating symptoms of disease. Providing relief of
symptoms is an important role for the physician, but
too rapid intervention can interfere with critical diagnostic or fundamental therapeutic measures. Patients with urgent abdominal emergencies may
insist on narcotic pain relief. Clinicians may be
tempted to relieve the symptoms before deciding on
the need for surgical intervention. The loss of mental alertness and the masking of physical signs produced by narcotics can make a decision on urgent
intervention even more difficult. Similarly, in situations of diagnostic uncertainty it may be essential
to document ischemia by doing an ECG even before
attempting to provide pain relief with nitroglycerin.
Thus, failure to institute timely intervention can
lead to errors of urgency, but so can well-inten-
tioned but premature symptomatic treatment. Clinicians have the difficult task of knowing when to
intervene before diagnosis and when to delay treating symptoms until treatment can be directed to the
underlying cause.

Even urgent conditions may require measured
gradual therapy, rather than heroic action. Many of
the most extreme physiologic problems produce
compensatory responses that make rapid correction
dangerous. Too rapid reheating in severe hypothermia may induce cardiac arrhythmias. Rapid restora-
tion of severe longstanding hypothyroidism may
induce cardiac decompensation or inadequate adre-
nal response. In other conditions individual organ
systems cannot adjust to abrupt changes in their
environment. Overly rapid correction of acidosis in
diabetic ketoacidosis may induce cellular edema in
the central nervous system. In other cases the therapy necessary to rapidly correct abnormalities is

more dangerous than the abnormality itself. Overly rapid parenteral replacement of potassium does not allow for intercellular transport and can lead to cardiac arrhythmia due to transient intravascular hyperkalemia.

Often after efforts to formulate an immediate clinical prognosis we conclude that the disease is potentially serious but treatment is not urgent. In this common situation it can often be extremely valuable to assess how this particular patient's disease is actually progressing. Many diseases follow a relatively constant rate of progression. Thus observation and careful measurement over a relatively short period of time often provide us with the best measure of the individual's actual prognosis. To accomplish these measurements we need what we will call a test of prognosis. For instance, tests of prognosis may involve sequential pulmonary function tests to determine whether sarcoidosis should be treated; repeat measurement of 24-hour urine protein to determine whether progressive renal disease is likely; or follow-up measurement of intraocular pressure to determine when intervention is indicated.

In summary, prediction, the first step in the therapeutic process, requires us to assess risk of disease and prognosis once disease develops. These predictions require a knowledge of the natural history of disease based on group risk and prognostic factors. Prognosis also requires us to incorporate what is known about the individual and the severity and urgency of the disease in developing an individual clinical prognosis. Adequate assessment of severity and urgency provides a basis for assessing the immediate consequences to the patient in the absence of treatment. Tests of prognosis on the individual often provide the best long-term measures of the individual's prognosis.

The world of medicine has changed enormously since the nineteenth century when the role of the physician was often to simply be with the patient while observing the natural history of disease. Yet it remains essential that clinicians understand the natural history of a disease in order to predict the risk of disease and the prognosis once a disease develops. Knowing when to intervene and when to leave well enough alone is now, as always, an important clinical skill. Once we have attempted to predict the course of disease in the absence of treatment, it is then possible to assess the advantages and disadvantages of instituting therapy.

# *8*

# *Effectiveness*

Having assessed the patient's risk of disease and prognosis once disease develops, clinicians are required to ask the question, "Could we do better?" For many conditions the process is self-limited, and the option to observe or help the patient deal temporarily with the symptoms is all that is necessary. When considering prescribing therapy, however, clinicians must address the questions of effectiveness. Is the treatment likely to help this particular patient? Increasingly the medical profession is also being asked to address the question, "Is this therapy cost-effective?"

How do we decide if a therapy is effective? Often we rely on official recommendations and select the "indicated treatment of choice." But where do these official recommendations come from? Decisions on the effectiveness of a therapy come from two basic sources, clinical research and clinical experience.

## CLINICAL RESEARCH

Well-designed, controlled clinical trials have become our gold standard for judging the efficacy of treatment for a well-defined group of patients with a well-defined disease. The use of control groups in controlled clinical trials provides a means of comparing a study therapy with the effects of placebo or standard therapy. The size of a well-designed study aims to ensure that when real, clinically important differences exist in larger populations, the investigation's samples will produce statistically significant results. Randomization of individuals to study and control groups helps ensure, at least in large trials, that the types of patients in the study and control groups will be very similar.*

Ideally, neither patients nor investigators in controlled clinical trials know whether the patient has been assigned to a study or control group. This double-blinding helps to ensure objective assessment of outcome free of the placebo effect. Careful follow-up limits the impact of loss–to–follow-up among those with poor outcomes. Any of these techniques, however, can be less than totally successful. Controlled clinical trials are not a panacea for the problems of judging effectiveness of therapy. The limitations of even well-designed and carefully-implemented studies include the:

Nonrandom selection of special types of patients for inclusion in an investigation.

Limited ability to predict the long-term and secondary efforts of therapy.

---

*Increased emphasis is being placed on the use of nonrandomized "outcome studies." These studies can, in theory, replace controlled clinical trials only if the prognostic factors that affect outcome are well known and are accurately measured in the study and control groups. In this situation some investigators believe that statistical adjustment can, in theory, replace randomization. Despite the cost savings inherent in this approach, it must be used very carefully or study results will be misleading due to unrecognized biases.*

## Nonrandom Selection of Patients

In controlled clinical trials, patients are not selected by chance from among all individuals. Patients are usually selected for studies because they are cooperative and compliant and are free of other illness or medication that is likely to interfere with or complicate the treatment or its assessment. High-risk groups are often excluded from controlled clinical trials. Children, pregnant women, and the elderly, for instance, are often excluded. The unique or particular characteristics of any one patient may alter the benefits they receive. Technically we speak of controlled clinical trials as being able to establish efficacy rather than effectiveness. Efficacy implies benefit in an investigation. Effectiveness implies benefit under the conditions of clinical care.

## Long-Term and Secondary Effects of a Therapy

In addition to the difficulty of extrapolating from controlled clinical trials, clinicians must recognize that controlled clinical trials follow patients' experiences over a defined and frequently relatively short period of time. Thus they cannot be expected to accurately assess the long-term or secondary effects of treatments. Secondary effects such as the eventual development of drug resistance may not be anticipated by even the most well-designed, controlled clinical trial. When treatments are applied to large numbers of individuals dynamic changes over time may occur that cannot be foreseen by the inherently static, or one-point-in-time, controlled clinical trials. The successful treatment of a sexually transmitted disease, for instance, may actually lead to an increased incidence of the disease by lowering the fear of the disease and reducing the precautions taken to prevent its occurrence.*

The dangers of extrapolating from controlled clinical trials should not discourage clinicians. It is impossible to practice medicine without extrapolating beyond the data. An awareness of the potentials for error inherent in this process, however, can help us maintain an analytical attitude and an open mind.

Controlled clinical trials rarely answer all the questions we must face clinically. If we know how to read between the lines of the official recommendations, we soon recognize the importance that even official recommendations place on clinical judgment based on clinical experience. Official recommendations rarely say "must;" they usually say "should," "may," or "can," indicating that considerable latitude exists for selecting a particular therapy. When recommendations say that therapy must be selected on a "case-by-case" basis, or "if clinically indicated" the meaning between the lines is . . . "there's no clear-cut answer. Use your clinical judgment." How do clinicians develop the necessary clinical judgment? Carefully observing the outcome of clinical decisions and learning from this experience is an indispensable component of medical decision-making.

## CLINICAL EXPERIENCE

Clinical experience often allows us to apply broad general lessons to new situations. In addition, when we speak of the benefits of experience, we often say that a doctor's clinical judgment is "tempered" by experience. What do we mean by that? Tempered by experience implies that a clinician has seen the good and the bad: the good and bad outcome, the

---

*As we will discuss in the chapter on safety, the limitations of controlled clinical trials are even greater when trying to assess safety.*

complicated and uncomplicated surgery, the common and not so common side effect. Experienced clinicians are often more realistic about the possibility of problems and more realistic about the potential for benefit. It is hoped that experience also teaches clinicians methods for avoiding the problems and increasing the chances of success. They know how to get the job done.

Clinical experience is an important basis for choosing therapy. Unfortunately, clinical experience needs to be critically examined before it can serve as a reliable means of judging the effectiveness of a therapy. Clinical experience has its inherent limitations. Enormous potential for drawing misleading conclusions exists when relying on our observation of the results of limited clinical experience. Sir William Osler wrote, "We are constantly misled by the ease with which our minds fall into the rut of one or two experiences"[4].

The tendency of clinicians to draw conclusions from limited experience is symbolized by the old medical story in which a physician who has seen one case proclaims "in my experience," while a physician who has seen two cases retorts "in my case series," only to be one upped by the physician with three cases who proclaims "again and again and again." Thus, to obtain maximum benefit from experience one must also recognize how it can lead us astray. Judging effectiveness based on experience is limited by:

The selection process that determines which patients a physician sees.
The selective follow-up that occurs after treatment.

## Patient Selection

The selection of patients we see may distort our experience due to limited numbers and types of patients seen. Any one clinician's quantity of experience is limited. Most clinicians will see only a small number of patients with a particular disease, and come to remember these patients as their prototype pattern of the disease. Specialization has been medicine's major method for overcoming the limited quantity of experience. Specialists, however, frequently see a special selection of patients. Specialists in our medical system usually see the more severe or difficult to diagnose cases of disease. For instance, seeing only patients with complications of duodenal ulcer disease, a gastroenterologist might easily conclude that a duodenal ulcer carries a poor prognosis and warrants intensive, invasive, and potentially dangerous therapy.

Generalists also can be misled by experience since patients tend to seek medical care when their symptoms are at their worst. Any clinician who has worked in an environment where there is some delay in scheduling nonemergency visits has heard patients say, "Wouldn't you know it, it's gone by the time I get to the doctor!" For chronic diseases this process also occurs as the disease symptoms wax and wane over time. If patients seek care at the point of maximum symptoms, any treatment, regardless of its effectiveness, may be associated with subsequent improvement. This phenomena, known as regression to the mean, can systematically affect the way clinicians view the effectiveness of their therapy.

## Selective Follow-Up

Learning from patients' responses to therapy can be misleading because:

The lack of controls may produce deceptively good
    results.

The results of the treatment itself often affect whether the patient returns for follow-up. Recall of experience is affected by the drama of the situation.

In controlled clinical trials the inclusion of a control group helps prevent bias in the assessment of outcome and also takes into account the placebo effect. The tendency to see what we expect to see or what we want to observe can have a profound effect on how we interpret the outcome of treatment. In clinical practice the placebo effect also distorts the assessment of outcome. The placebo effect is a powerful phenomena in which biologically inert treatments have been experimentally demonstrated to produce real objective changes in 30 percent or more of patients receiving the placebo. The pattern of response to placebos typically resembles the pharmacologic response to active drugs. Placebo responses are not limited to the patient's subjective experiences; placebos alter laboratory values and other measures of objective physiology.

In addition to the selective sampling and biased assessment of experience, problems may result from selective follow-up and recall of experience. Attempts to learn by follow-up of individual patients are complicated by the fact that follow-up is not a chance phenomenon. For instance, dissatisfied and disappointed patients may be disproportionately represented among those who are lost to follow-up. If only those who are satisfied or alternatively only those who are dissatisfied return, clinicians gain a distorted perception of their therapeutic experience.

The human ability to recall experience is not primarily a function of frequency. Memory is closely linked with emotion and drama. The more personal the reaction to the patient, and the more dramatic the patient's problem, the more easily the patient and the disease are remembered and recalled. The patient who dies, the mistaken diagnosis, the furious attending, all raise the ability to recall regardless of the representativeness of the situations. The great eighteenth century clinician Heberden pointed out that "new medicines and methods of cure always work miracles for a while"[4]. Recent improvement in assessing effectiveness helps ensure that not too many apparent miracles come along every year. The individual physician must still maintain a healthy skepticism about the effectiveness of therapies.

## COST-EFFECTIVENESS

Increasingly, the medical profession is being called on to assess more than effectiveness. We are being asked to assess cost effectiveness of therapies, especially new therapies. Today, physicians practice in an environment where technology is changing rapidly, and we are constantly tantalized by the allure of modern technology. Each new issue of the most respected journals and each new grand rounds by the most acclaimed expert bring to light new ways to treat patients. How could any physician help but be impressed with the newest technology-producing images from living patients that remind us of textbook pictures previously available only at surgery or autopsy?

In an earlier era, many of the advances in medical technology were accompanied and restrained by an element of risk to the patient. Coronary catheterization had the small risk of causing a stroke or myocardial infarction. Liver and kidney biopsy held the risk of bleeding. Thus, despite these techniques' usefulness in specific circumstances, physicians had a reason to be restrained in their use. No such restraint need accompany the newest generation of medical miracles. Magnetic resonance imaging and echocardiography not only can be done without invading the body, but are believed to be free of the dangers attributed to radiation. If they were free of cost, their use could be justified for nearly every patient on every visit. Thus we are confronted with a new reality. Increasingly, the seductive effects of technology are only constrained by the costs, not by the risk to the patient.

New technology has become one of the major driving forces behind the increased cost of medical care, which is now well over ten percent of the gross national product. The implications of the cost of medical care are just beginning to be felt by the individual clinician. In the past, new therapies were used whenever there was evidence of effectiveness. Thus physicians felt an obligation to implement any therapy in which there was any net benefit to the patient. Physicians have often sought to do everything possible rather than everything proven.

Rarely were treatments compared to each other to determine which was the most effective. Rather, individual clinicians, with the advice of individual experts, were expected to weigh the advantages and disadvantages of alternative therapies, usually without regard to cost. Cost considerations were left to the administrator and the economist since most patients felt protected by third party insurance. The word cost, however, is increasingly being added to the word effectiveness. When the two words are combined often enough, they become nearly synonymous. Thus, it is important for the individual clinician to appreciate what cost-effectiveness means and the ways it can mislead us.

## Analysis of Cost-Effectiveness

Formal analysis of cost-effectiveness produces a cost-effectiveness ratio. The cost-effectiveness ratio

compares the costs as measured in dollars\* divided
by the effectiveness of care as measured in what
economists call quality adjusted life years (QALYS).
One QALY represents one additional year of full health for one person, the average person who is to receive the therapy. One QALY implies the difference
between death, which is usually set at 0, and the
previous state of health, which is usually set at 1, for
this hypothetical average person. Thus a QALY may
be thought of as one year of life saved for one typical individual receiving the therapy.

In calculating a cost-effective ratio economists
calculate the net costs of the therapy (cost minus
any savings from reduced complications) for providing the therapy to all eligible patients divided by the
number of additional QALYS that result. The resulting cost-effectiveness ratio is an estimate of the average number of dollars that need to be spent to
produce one additional year of life for one typical
individual. Economists have found that some of our
most successful interventions, such as treatment of
severe hypertension, cost well under $10,000 per
QALY. They have found, however, that much of what
is routinely done as part of medical care costs in the
range of $10,000 to $25,000 per QALY. Recently the
costs of new advances in medical care have often
produced costs per QALY in the $25,000 to $100,000
range or more.

In dealing with the concept of cost-effectiveness,
it is important that clinicians recognize that after
all the cost calculations are done the judgment of
whether it is worth it still needs to be made. In
asking whether it is worth it, clinicians must
appreciate the use of three different terms in
cost-effective analysis:

---

\**Which costs to include and how to take into account costs that occur
at a later date have been a controversial issue. Cost-effectiveness analysis is often done in terms of the cost to society, thus including all
medical care costs regardless of who pays the bills.*

Cost savings
Cost effective
More and most cost effective

Failure to appreciate the meaning of these terms may lead to some important errors in their application. Cost savings implies that money is saved, that the actual cost of care is reduced. This reduction may be due to more efficient or effective therapy that reduces the cost of achieving the same benefit or even greater benefit. Almost everyone would agree that cost-saving measures make sense whether they are achieved by new forms of therapy, such as lithotripsy, or new ways to deliver existing therapy, such as selective use of outpatient surgery.

Cost effective as opposed to cost savings may mean one of two very different things. Cost effective often implies that a new technology or approach to therapy has been assessed in terms of costs and benefits, and the additional benefit gained is considered worth the cost. Increasingly, "worth the cost" implies that it fits into the ballpark figures that have presented for existing forms of therapy.

Cost effective may also have an entirely different meaning. It may imply that the new approach produces a reduction in benefits, but that the reduced benefits are worth the reduced costs. For clinicians, this distinction is important. In theory, it implies that cost-effectiveness analysis can be used to decide how to increase the benefits while minimizing the increase in cost, or it can be used to decide how to reduce the costs while minimizing the reduction in benefits. Thus clinicians must recognize that cost effective and maximum benefit to the patient are not synonymous.

Most cost effective often implies that more than one therapeutic option for the same condition has been compared, and one has been found to cost less per QALY saved than the other(s). It is important to recognize, however, that when one therapy is found to be the most cost effective, it does not necessarily exclude use of other therapies as well. For instance, if we are comparing the cost effectiveness of angioplasty versus coronary artery bypass surgery, or lithotripsy versus surgical removal of stones, we will find that angioplasty and lithotripsy are more cost effective than surgical therapies. The finding of more or most cost effective may imply that when the two options are equally applicable, lithotripsy and angioplasty are indicated. There will still be individual cases, however, when the two therapies need to be combined, or when the surgical therapy is substantially more effective so that it is considered worth the additional cost.

American medicine often has the luxury to not only choose between therapies, but also to combine therapies, allowing additional treatment when one therapy is unsuccessful. Thus the finding that one therapy is more or most cost effective does not imply that the less cost-effective treatment should be discarded.

## Cost Effectiveness in Practice

New technologies, including new drugs, are often introduced and paid for in medical practice after their effectiveness has been established only for a specific disease or treatment. These "indications" are part of the formal approval process that the Food and Drug Administration applies to new drugs and more recently to major changes in medical technology. The new technology is often a substantial improvement over existing technology when used for the narrowly defined approved indication. Even if it is expensive the new technology may be cost effective. That is, the additional expenditure may be worth the additional expense. Once technology is introduced into practice, it is common for physicians to begin to extend the indications and apply the technology to new clinical situations. In these new situations, the technology may still be useful but often it no longer represents a major advance. Often, in fact, the new technology is used in addition to, rather than as a replacement for, the older methods. Thus, frequently, it merely adds to the expense without adding to the information. In addition, the widespread diffusion of expensive technology has often meant that each institution used its equipment only a small percentage of the time.

Once a drug or technology is approved by the Food and Drug Administration, physicians have the right to use the treatment for purposes beyond the approved indications. Thus, it is not unusual to see drugs and other technologies used for conditions other than the approved indication. Often those indications such as propranolol for thyrotoxicosis or amitriptyline for peripheral neuropathy have extensive, favorable clinical experience, but the manufacturers have not gone to the expense of securing Food and Drug Administration approval for these indications. Remember, however, that drug or other technology that is effective and approved for one indication may or may not be effective for another.

Similarly, it is important to recognize that once a technology has been established as cost effective for one indication, it does not automatically imply that it will continue to be cost effective as the indications expand or the way the therapy is delivered changes. Cost effectiveness for one indication does not imply that the therapy itself is cost effective. For instance, imagine that lithotripsy has been shown to be cost effective for treating kidney stones less than 2 cm when used as a substitute for surgery. It is possible that lithotripsy will be used to treat all patients with kidney stones less than 2 cm as soon as

the disease is identified. In this new use lithotripsy
may not be cost effective, or worth the cost, since
the vast majority of stones pass spontaneously without the need for surgery. Thus, it is important that
clinicians understand the meaning of the terms cost
savings, cost effective, and most cost effective.*
Only by appreciating the meaning of the terms can
we expect to recognize that cost effective may be
used to mean that reduced benefits are worth the
reduced cost, that the most cost-effective therapy
may not be the only therapy that should be used,
and that cost-effectiveness for one indication does
not make the therapy itself cost effective.

Having explored the issues and problems posed by
the clinician's need to deal with effectiveness and
cost effectiveness, let us turn our attention to the
issue of safety.

---

**The terminology cost savings is also used more generically than it has
been used in this chapter to indicate reduced cost without regard to the
change in effectiveness. When assessing the most cost-effect therapy
economists also use the concept of incremental or marginal cost-effectiveness ratio to measure the additional cost of achieving additional
QALYS.

# 9

# *Safety*

"There are some patients whom we cannot help: there are none whom we cannot harm" wrote Bloomfield[5], emphasizing the importance of paying particular attention to safety. Yet in recent years iatrogenic or doctor-induced disease has become one of the major reasons for hospital admissions. In fact it was at the top of the list of avoidable and reversible diseases among medical admissions in at least one study[6].

Decisions on therapy require more than an assessment of the effectiveness of therapy; they require an assessment of the safety of therapy followed by an effort to weigh the potential benefits against the potential risks.

Known risks of therapy can be characterized using two basic features:

Probability of side effects
Severity of side effects

Recognition and anticipation of these features of safety help us minimize medical mistakes.

## PROBABILITY OF SIDE EFFECTS

Assessing the probability of an adverse effect is aided by knowledge of the therapy, the patient, and the interactions that occur. Knowledge of a therapy's mechanism of action may help in determining the probability of an adverse effect. Some drug side effects are so closely linked to the mechanism of action that they are really expected effects of the drug. Doctors and patients should not be surprised by their occurrence. Warfarin in therapeutic doses produces easy bruisability and potentially dangerous bleeding due to its therapeutic effect on the coagulation system. Other drugs exert metabolic effects that are a natural by-product of their mechanism of action. Thiazide diuretics can be expected to lower serum potassium levels, while spirolactone and triamterene can be expected to raise potassium levels.

Drugs with a small margin of safety between their therapeutic and toxic levels can be expected to have a high probability of adverse effects. Special care must be taken to monitor these drugs and detect side effects early. Digoxin and lithium are examples of drugs in which doses only moderately above the usual levels can produce adverse effects. With some drugs such as dilantin, a small increase in dose may produce a dramatic increase in blood levels once protein binding of the drug is maximal. Patients should be specifically instructed to watch for the nausea of digoxin toxicity, the tremor of lithium, and the ataxia of phenytoin overdose. Judicious use of blood-level monitoring can aid in the dosage adjustment for many of these drugs.

Not recognizing which patients have a high probability of adverse effects leads to many medical mistakes. Patients with limited or altered ability to handle drugs include the very young and the elderly. They are at greater risk of adverse effects due to their reduced ability to metabolize and excrete medications. Standard doses of digoxin, cimetidine, aminoglycosides, and lithium, for instance, can be toxic in a healthy elderly individual whose renal function has declined, even in the absence of known renal disease. Even in the presence of similar blood levels the elderly may have increased sensitivity to many drug effects and thus often can be treated effectively with low dosages. Such drugs as benzodiazepines, warfarin, aminoglycosides, and quinidine are more likely to be toxic in the elderly and patients with underlying disease that affects metabolism or excretion.

Renal and hepatic disease often affects an individual's sensitivity to drugs. Much attention has been directed to the effects of reduced renal function on the dosage of digoxin and aminoglycosides. In the presence of substantial renal dysfunction, however, a long list of drugs requires dosage adjustment. Impaired hepatic function poses a danger when drugs are metabolized or excreted via the liver. Day-to-day fluctuation in the ability of the liver to metabolize drugs can be great, especially in the millions of Americans who drink enough alcohol to induce hepatic enzymes. When sober, these individuals' livers have increased metabolic potential. When drinking actively their metabolic activity falls dramatically, leaving them susceptible to toxic effects. Failure to recognize a high probability of adverse effects often means that the physician fails to alter the dose, avoid the drug, or make efforts to recognize side effects early.

Administration of multiple drugs increases the probability of drug interactions. Drugs may interact if one drug changes the metabolism of another drug, alters absorption, blocks the manifestation of another drug's side effects, or by a variety of other mechanisms. The potential for drug interaction is nearly unlimited. Drugs known to alter the hepatic blood flow, such as cimetadine, or alter hepatic metabolic activity, such as barbiturates, frequently affect the action of other drugs and cause complicated interactions. Drugs such as antacids and cholestyramine may interfere with absorption of other drugs. When added to a medical regimen their timing should be spaced as distantly as possible from other drugs, and their potential for affecting absorption should be appreciated. Particularly dangerous side effects can occur when one medication blocks the manifestation of another drug's side effects. Beta blockers, especially propranolol, may block the hunger, nervousness, and other epinephrine-mediated manifestations of hypoglycemia, leaving the patient with only sweating as an early clinical manifestation of hypoglycemia.

The number of interactions expands geometrically and occurs in difficult to anticipate directions as the number of drugs administered increases. Thus, it is important to keep the number of drugs at a minimum. In addition to considering the probability of side effects, it is important to consider the severity of the side effects.

## SEVERITY OF SIDE EFFECTS

The severity of a side effect is determined by a number of features, including:

Its potential for morbidity and mortality
Whether it can be easily detected and reversed
When it will occur

The severity of side effects depends on the type of harm that may occur. Side effects such as pulmonary emboli secondary to birth control pills may be of great concern because of their life-threatening potential in a young woman, despite the low probability of occurrence. Thus, failure to take into account serious but low-probability side effects, such as aplastic anemia secondary to drugs like chloramphenicol and butazolidine, or anaphylaxis secondary to IV radiology-contrast materials become important mistakes.

The severity of a side effect depends in part on how easily the side effect can be detected and how easily it can be reversed if detected. Drugs that cause depression (such as methyldopa, propranolol, and reserpine) can be especially dangerous because the effects may be subtle and unrecognized initially by the patient or the doctor. The consequences of these drugs can often be avoided by warning the patient of the effects and carefully monitoring the patient, looking for signs of depression.

The reversibility of these side effects means that their severity can be reduced by careful follow-up. Other treatment complications may not be so reversible. An emboli dislodged during an invasive procedure may have irreversible effects, yet early detection of most procedural complications (such as a bowel perforation, arrythmias, or bleeding) can often reduce the severity of the complication.

The severity of a side effect is also dependent on when it will occur. Often long-term risks such as cancer may be less serious in an elderly person than short-term risks such as increased congestive heart failure. An immediate risk of arrhythmia when the patient is being closely observed on cardiac monitor may be much less serious than a lesser risk of arrhythmia a week after hospital discharge.

Knowing when a side effect may occur allows physicians to take steps to reduce the severity and consequences of the reaction. Despite potential severity of anaphylaxis due to IM penicillin, the fact that it occurs less than an hour after administration allows physicians to take precautions to reduce the consequences. At times this requires careful instructions for patients. Prazasin is particularly prone to hypotension with the initial administration. Taking the first dose before bed and warning the patient to remain lying down for several hours after initial use usually prevents serious consequences.

Considering the timing of the adverse effect is also important to reduce the severity of side effects that occur on sudden withdrawal. Withdrawal of addicting drugs such as narcotics, barbiturates, or alcohol can often create problems that may first come to light when the patient is admitted to the hospital for another reason. Even worse are rebound symptoms. Clonidine rebound, for instance, is characterized by severe hypertension that is often difficult to control. Sudden discontinuation of phenytoin, phenobarbital, or other anticonvulsant drugs can produce status epilepticus. Beta-blocker rebound may result in unstable angina or even myocardial infarction.

Failure to consider the severity of a potential side effect by taking into account the potential for morbidity and mortality, the ease of detection and reversibility, and the timing of the side effect can lead to many medical mistakes. Recognition of the probability and severity of known side effects can go a long way toward minimizing the occurrence of these predictable risks.

## UNPREDICTABLE RISKS

Some risks are not known to the medical profession and thus cannot easily be anticipated. Unknown side effects occur when they have not been previously reported or recognized. Clinicians need to be especially alert for the occurrence of unknown side effects whenever they deal with recently approved or inadequately studied therapies.

Since the days of the thalidomide tragedy, most American physicians have come to believe that approval of a drug by the Food and Drug Administration implies safety or at least clearly-defined and well-understood side effects. Unfortunately even controlled clinical trials that are adequate for demonstrating the efficacy of a therapy are often inadequate for assessing safety. For rare but serious side effects of therapy large numbers of patients are required before one can expect to observe the side effect. Imagine for instance that one wished to detect the occurrence of penicillin anaphylaxis, which occurs an average once per 10,000 uses. It would require 30,000 patients to receive IM penicillin to have a 95 percent probability of observing at least one case of penicillin anaphylaxis. To have a 95 percent probability of finding at least one case of chloramphenicol-induced, irreversible aplastic anemia, which occurs approximately once in 50,000 uses, one would need to observe 150,000 patients receiving chloramphenicol. This principle, known as the rule of three, reminds us that safety cannot be assumed, even when no adverse effects have been observed. Thus it is not surprising that the antibiotic chloramphenicol was widely and casually used in the United States for over a decade before irreversible aplastic anemia was recognized as a rare but serious side effect. The use of this antibiotic for common bacterial or even viral infections led to a large number of deaths due to aplastic anemia, despite the fact that this complication occurs only once in many thousands of uses. Systematic surveillance and skepticism of new drugs by individual physicians is necessary if this type of idiosyncratic reaction is to be recognized and rapidly dealt with in the future.

Unrecognized effects of treatments are especially likely when the therapy has not been well studied. This can occur when established drugs are used for

new indications or over-the-counter "natural" therapies, such as vitamins and minerals, are used for
treating disease. For several decades after vitamin D
was recognized as necessary to prevent rickets, the
public and many physicians regarded it as safe and
useful even in high doses. Its widespread use at
high doses resulted in considerable morbidity before
the medical community fully accepted the dangers
to the kidneys, brain, bones, and arteries, which
vitamin D overdoses can produce.

Women who may be pregnant require special precautions. The dangers of drugs during pregnancy
have been increasingly appreciated by most clinicians. The rule of regarding all drugs as dangerous
during pregnancy is unfortunately a good rule-of-
thumb because of how little is known about the effects of drugs during pregnancy. Animal testing has
been shown to be an unreliable guide since ter-
atogenic effects in one animal species often do not
predict effects in other species. Many drugs are the-
oretically the most dangerous during the early
weeks of pregnancy, at the time when a woman is
not aware of her pregnancy. This makes avoidance
of exposure a very difficult job. Every woman
placed on a drug should be specifically questioned
about her last menstrual period and use of birth
control. Women who are attempting to get pregnant
should be encouraged to avoid all but essential medications. These precautions can help avoid many
medication risks during pregnancy.

Errors in recognizing and minimizing the dangers
of treatment are important and frequently preventable sources of poor therapeutic outcomes. Having
looked at principles of effectiveness and safety let
us turn our attention to how we combine benefits
and risks as part of therapeutic decision making.

# 10

# *Therapeutic Decisions*

The process of making therapeutic decisions consists of two conceptually separate but closely intertwined steps:

Developing and communicating a clinician's recommendation

Engaging the patient in informed consent

When an important step like major surgery is involved, these steps may be relatively elaborate and formalized by the signing of a written document. However, these two steps are part of even the briefest clinical encounter. Even when the physician says "this is what you should do" and the patient does it, a recommendation and consent are implied even if the recommendation is not explicitly communicated and the patient's consent is not explicitly obtained. Thus therapeutic decision making involves two distinct processes. Failure to recognize the existence of two separate processes is the source of frequent problems.

At one extreme, physicians assume they know best and believe their recommendations should be accepted by the patients without an independent analysis. These physicians often feel threatened by second opinions, feel challenged when patients ask prying questions, and feel they can't take care of patients if their recommendations are rejected.

At the other extreme are a growing number of physicians who adopt the attitude that their job is to convey the facts and not to provide an opinion. These physicians lay out the facts but make no recommendation. Patients have difficulties with this type of physician as well since they often are not engaged in the process, refuse to take responsibility, and fail to convey a special professional competence needed for a successful doctor-patient relationship.

There are patients who seek and accept these two types of physicians, but increasingly the competent physician is one who can accomplish both processes: Making therapeutic recommendations and engaging the patient in informed consent.

Let us begin by outlining the essential factors that clinicians must consider when developing a therapeutic recommendation. Then we will discuss the process of informed consent and see how these same factors must be considered by the patient.

## CLINICIAN'S RECOMMENDATION

When discussing safety we looked at two basic features that characterized safety: probability and severity. These same features can be used to characterize effectiveness as well. Thus, in theory, the task for the physician in developing a therapeutic decision is to compare the probability and severity of each potential therapy's effectiveness or benefits versus its adverse effects or risks. How can physicians approach this complex process called risk-benefit analysis? Often we start and stop by concentrating on the probability of occurrence of the benefits and the risks. When adequate and relevant data are available from controlled clinical trials, it is possible to compare these risks and benefits using a summary measurement known as the number-needed-to-treat.

In order to calculate a number-needed-to-treat we will assume that those in the treatment group have a better prognosis than those in the control group, the number-needed-to-treat for benefits is calculated as follows:

$$\frac{1}{\text{Probability of a good outcome in the treatment group} \quad - \quad \text{Probability of a good outcome in the control group}}$$

If study data are available that tell us that in a treatment group the probability of a good outcome with treatment is 3 in 5, while in a similar control group the probability of a good outcome without treatment is 2 in 5, the number-needed-to-treat for benefits is calculated as follows:

$$\frac{1}{\frac{3}{5} \quad - \quad \frac{2}{5}} = 5$$

This calculation tells us that five similar individuals on average need to be treated to obtain one additional good outcome. The number-needed-to-treat may be used to compare different treatments or to compare the benefits of a treatment to the risks of the treatment.*

*When using the number-needed-to-treat to compare treatments, however, we must be careful to realize that studies treat patients for differing lengths of time. It is possible, however, to take into account how long a patient was treated and compare treatments on a comparable basis.*

The number-needed-to-treat for adverse effects or risk is calculated as follows:

$$\frac{1}{\text{Probability of the adverse effect in the treated group} - \text{Probability of the adverse effect in the untreated group}}$$

Thus if an adverse effect occurs twice in 100 among a treated group and the same effect occurs once in 100 among a control group, then the number-needed-to-treat for risk equals:

$$\frac{1}{\frac{2}{100} - \frac{1}{100}} = 100$$

A number-needed-to-treat for the benefits and a parallel number-needed-to-treat for the adverse effects or risks can be obtained. The number-needed-to-treat for benefits tells us on average how many individuals need to be prescribed the therapy to produce one additional good outcome, such as preventing a myocardial infarction. Similarly, the number-needed-to-treat for risk tells us how many individuals need to be prescribed the therapy to produce one additional adverse outcome, such as a stroke. If the number-needed-to-treat for benefit (prevention of myocardial infarction) is 5, while the risk number needed to treat for adverse effects (stroke) is 100, then we know that the benefit is 20 times as likely to occur as the adverse risk. Often that's all we need to know to make a recommendation, especially if a stroke and a myocardial infarction are considered equally severe outcomes that occur about the same time.

Frequently, however, the process is more complicated. Physicians are usually forced to rely not on objective data from investigations but upon a subjective or perceived assessment of probability. In addition, the perceived severity and timing of the potential outcomes often differ and these differences need to be taken into consideration. Perceived probability implies an educated guess based on what is known from the literature about groups of individuals who receive a therapy, as well as what is known about the individual patient. Perceived severity is also called utility. Utility implies that a particular outcome is not viewed as equally good or equally bad by everyone. The loss of a leg, blindness, or even a stroke may have different perceived severity or utility to different individuals.

In order to reach a recommendation on therapy we need to combine estimates of perceived probability and perceived severity. This may be done quantitatively using a technique known as decision analysis.* More commonly this is done qualitatively and often almost unconsciously without focusing on the component parts of the decision.

Whose perceptions should we be using in developing a therapeutic recommendation, our own or those of the patient? In theory we should be doing our best to incorporate the patient's probabilities and utilities into our recommendations. This, however, may be difficult. Ultimately, the patient's own assessment of the probabilities and utilities is what matters and is what we deal with in the process of informed consent.

In accomplishing the separate process of therapeutic recommendation and informed consent, clinicians alone and then clinicians and patients together

---

*In decision analysis a probability and a utility are estimated for each potential outcome of a therapeutic option. The probability scores (0 to 1) and the utility scores (usually 0 = death, 1 = full health) for each outcome are then multipled together. These expected utilities for each potential outcome of a particular therapy are added together to produce an overall expected utility for the therapeutic option. Using these numbers, it is possible to compare the overall expected utility of one therapy to another.

must struggle with the same two basic features—
perceived probabilities and perceived severity or
utility. Let us turn our attention to the process of informed consent. We will look at the requirements of
the process and then see how we can avoid many
mistakes in the dual processes of developing and
communicating a therapeutic recommendation and
engaging a patient in informed consent.

## INFORMED CONSENT

Informed consent has been codified by law and professional standards to require three criteria:

Capacity to decide
Pertinent information
Uncoerced decision making

In order to engage in the process, patients need to
have the capacity to decide. This is not the same as
legal competence. Rather capacity to decide implies
that a patient can understand and participate in the
process. According to the President's Commission
on Bioethics, decision-making capacity requires a
set of stable values and goals; the ability to understand and communicate information; and the ability
to reason and to deliberate about one's choices[7].
Thus the capacity to decide implies that the patient
has the mental capacity to understand and communicate choices, rationally manipulate information,
and appreciate the situation and its consequences
for his or her life. In other words patients must be
able to engage in the intellectual work required to
make a decision. Often this step occurs instantly
since patients can be presumed to have the capacity
to decide unless there is strong evidence to the contrary.

Assuming a patient is capable of engaging in the process of informed consent, he or she needs to be informed of the essential elements that go into the decision process. Informed consent implies that doctors will walk the patient through the essential steps that they have taken in reaching their recommendation. This is done to ensure that the patient has the pertinent information and freely agrees. Defining what is pertinent information for the patient to be told has been a challenge for physicians and for the court system. Mazur[8] described three standards the courts have used. Initially, and in some states today, the courts adopted a professional-oriented standard that says that a physician should disclose to a patient what his or her peers in good standing disclose to their patients. In recent years, most courts have used the reasonable-person standard (or objective, patient-oriented standards) requiring physicians to convey what a reasonable person in the patient's position would want to know. A few courts have recently begun to apply a subjective patient-oriented standard requiring clinicians to disclose all that a particular patient would have wanted to know.

In the face of conflicting and difficult-to-define standards, the individual physician may have great difficulty deciding what information to disclose. These problems can usually be resolved by asking ourselves what information we used in evaluating the different options and reaching our own recommendation. Conveying this information and, in addition, responding to a patient's questions seem a reasonable compromise. Specifically, this pertinent information should include:

The rationale for therapy—the prognosis without therapy and a discussion of the reasons that therapy is being recommended.

The major benefit(s) expected from the therapy, including how the patient's own situation may alter
the probabilities for achieving the benefit.
The major risks of the treatment, including the probability, severity, and timing of these risks.
A description of the alternative therapeutic options
available and the degree of uncertainty with respect to the potential outcomes.

This pertinent information allows the patient to
actively evaluate the clinician's reasoning process. A
description of the major risks and benefits of the
recommended therapy allows the patient to develop
his or her own probabilities and utilities. A description of the other therapeutic options available allows
the patient to weigh the risks and benefits of alternative therapies.

Given this pertinent information, the patient
needs to be able to freely use the data and freely
make the decision. An uncoerced decision implies
that the decision to proceed with a therapy is ultimately the patient's. Lack of coercion means that
clinicians have done their best not to convey the
data to patients in ways that bias information or
overtly or subtly attempt to influence the decision.
Lack of coercion also implies that the decision-making process is free of the threat of consequences, including the threat to withhold medical care. Even
when clinicians cannot accept a patient's choice,
they have an obligation to refer patients to a source
of care if the care can be provided legally. Thus, informed consent implies that the patient has the capacity, data, and freedom to decide.

When clinicians make recommendations and patients make choices there are a number of sources
of medical mistakes. These problems come most obviously to light during the process of informed consent. It is helpful to use the framework of informed
consent to analyze the types of problems that occur.

Initially we will assume that the patient is competent to decide and start with the criteria of pertinent information. We will look at how doctors and patients often have different perceptions of probability and place different utilities on the outcome. We will also look at how a third factor, which we will call risk-taking attitudes, often influences decision making. Then we will look at the criteria of uncoerced decision making and see how consciously or unconsciously clinicians may use subtle coercion to influence the decision making process. Finally, we will return to the issue of patient capacity to decide and look at what can get in the way of patients' use of their capacity to decide.

## Pertinent Information: Perceived Probabilities

Doctors' and patients' perceptions of the probability of benefits and risks are often judged by the ease with which the benefits or risks can be imagined. Doctors and patients frequently confuse the probability of adverse effect with the ease of imaging their occurrence. Clinicians who have just taken care of a patient who died at surgery, suffered a complication of a procedure, or an adverse effect of a drug, quite understandably overestimate its probability of recurrence. In addition, clinicians often suffer from what has been called the gamblers fallacy, believing that chance runs in streaks or if you've seen a good outcome once you'll see a good outcome again soon. Just as clinicians may be biased by the ease of imagining a particular outcome, patients are also strongly influenced by the same effect. Patients who have a frieı. ' or family member who died of Hodgkin's disease or heart disease may be better able to envision the risks and benefits, but are also more likely to overestimate the probabilities of a bad outcome.

It is very difficult for doctors and patients to gain an accurate, perceived probability for rare events. Usually the probability of rare events, those occurring less than one or two times per 100, are either overestimated or underestimated. Thus, when confronted with the probability of death from routine surgery or a life-threatening complication of medications, both doctors and patients may overestimate the probability of occurrence. Alternatively, they may put it out of their minds as too remote and too horrible to contemplate, thus underestimating the probability.

How can patients and clinicians gain more accurate perceptions? There are several methods that help.

1. The number-needed-to-treat approach provides a method of making research data more easily accessible. If 2000 asymptomatic middle-aged men need to be treated with aspirin before one additional man will experience a cerebral bleed, while 100 such individuals need to be treated before one myocardial infarction is prevented, these numbers needed to treat provide an understandable means of expressing complicated data about rare events.
2. When dealing with small risks in the range of one to five percent it may be more accurate to speak in terms of odds instead of probabilities. By odds we mean the chances favoring an event versus the chances against an event. Thus instead of a two percent probability we might speak of odds of 1:49 (or rounded to 1:50). When the probability is four percent instead of two percent it may be difficult to perceive the difference. However, the odds are now 1:24 instead of 1:49, a difference that is often easier to appreciate. By using odds instead of probabilities doctors and patients are often

able to deal more accurately with relatively rare events.

3. A commonly used means of conveying rare events is to compare the risk to the risk of occurrence of events in everyday experience. Thus clinicians may use or abuse expressions like "you're more likely to be run over crossing the street, or dying from a heart attack." These expressions can be helpful if accurate. Clinicians, however, need to recognize that risks like dying from an auto accident or heart attack may be high, but this risk is spread over a lifetime, while the risks of the therapy are usually more immediate.

Thus it is a common mistake for doctors and patients to have unrealistic perceptions of probabilities. Efforts to help patients understand the numbers and relate them to life experiences can help to make estimates of probability more nearly accurate.

## Pertinent Information: Utilities

Utilities imply that a particular outcome has different meaning or value to different individuals. The acceptability of life with varying degrees or different types of disability is an important consideration, especially for complex decisions. The decision for dialysis versus kidney transplant, medical versus surgical management of coronary artery disease, or chemotherapy versus observation for metastatic cancer may well tilt one way or the other, depending on how doctors and patients weigh the utility of different forms of disability.

Patients, and at times doctors, may suffer from what may be called the dread effect. The dread effect is a powerful force that results in overestimation of the severity (and sometimes the probability) of a particular outcome. Life without a leg, with a colostomy, or after a mastectomy may seem unbearable. Fortunately, the dread effect is often relatively easy to bring under control by having patients verbalize their fears. Often talking with other patients who live happy and productive lives after losing a leg, having a colostomy, or mastectomy is enough to convert the dread effect into a realistic concern.

In addition to different utilities placed on the same outcome, doctors and patients often differ in how they value or place utilities on time. Living a year may seem like half as long as two years to a doctor. To a patient, that first year may be worth much more than the second year. This is especially true if it allows the patient to get his or her affairs in order, see friends or family, or make a special trip. In addition, patients may appropriately focus more on the quality of remaining life than the quantity. Life spent in pain or in the hospital may not be valued as highly as a shorter life span of productivity or enjoyment. Thus the utilities placed on particular outcomes and the value of time may be very different for doctors and patients. Clinicians' failure to appreciate these differences leads to many errors in therapeutic decision making.

## Pertinent Information: Risk-Taking Attitudes

Ideally, a physician's recommendation is based on perceived probability and perceived severity. When these factors favor a therapy, the physician in theory recommends the treatment. Often, however, the physician's risk-taking attitude influences the recommendation, and the patient's risk-taking attitude influences how he or she reaches a decision.

Most clinicians express their desire to be risk neutral. That is, they favor taking action only when their combination of perceived probability and utility of the benefits outweigh those of the risk.* Few human beings, doctors included, are actually risk neutral. Most people fear the rare but catastrophic downside. They buy insurance to protect themselves from large risks even though they guarantee themselves a small financial loss in the form of an insurance premium. We will call this risk-aversive behavior. Alternatively, in the right situation many people may be risk seekers. They are willing to take a guaranteed small loss in exchange for a very small probability of a large gain, even though the odds are stacked against them. Witness the popularity of gambling. A particular individual may be a risk seeker or risk aversive depending on the circumstances.

In parallel with buying insurance and gambling are two common clinical situations where patients or clinicians or both have strong tendencies to deviate from risk neutrality. Failure to appreciate these situations may be important sources of error.

Patients are likely to be risk aversive in situations outside their control where there is a small but perceptible probability of an outcome of high perceived severity. Thus, most people fear airplane accidents even more than auto accidents. Similarly, many patients and nonsurgeons fear surgery out of proportion to the risk. The small but perceptable probability of an outcome such as interoperative death or postoperative pulmonary emboli may produce a risk-aversive patient. These patients and doctors often prefer a medical treatment more under their control and less likely to produce these rare but catastrophic downside risks. Thus doctors and patients may be risk aversive due to what we will call the insurance effect.

*\*When quantitating risk, risk neutral implies that once one obtains an overall expected utility for each therapeutic option, one will accept the therapeutic option with the largest overall expected utility.*

The anxiety produced by not knowing if and not knowing when may be more than the patient or the doctor is willing to bear. Clinicians, however, can influence the magnitude and consequences of the insurance effect and at times help to encourage patients to be less risk aversive. This can be done by providing patients with means to gain control by anticipating and minimizing the risks. Patients who know that early ambulation can reduce pulmonary emboli and who also feel they don't need to be in bed long after surgery will be less influenced by the insurance effect. Patients who stop smoking or lose weight before surgery not only reduce their risk but gain control by involvement in the process.

Some patients find that a low tolerance for risk causes them to favor the known status quo rather than the unknown effects of therapy. It is, of course, the patient's prerogative to be risk aversive. Individuals differ considerably in their tendency to be influenced by the insurance effect. Some patients actually prefer those forms of therapy that are outside their control, with a small probability of severe complication. They may then be able to escape the burden of taking responsibility for participating in a therapeutic process that may require them to change long-standing behaviors. Thus two individuals with the same perceived probabilities and perceived severity may select different treatments based on their risk-taking attitudes.

A second common situation, where doctors and patients are often not risk neutral, occurs when patients find themselves slipping away from their accustomed and desired state of health. When disease has progressed and therapy has not had its desired effects, patients are particularly likely to gamble or be risk seekers. Doctors and patients, like football quarterbacks, often "go for the longshot" when they perceive that time is running out. The football analogy may well propel many heroic efforts that have little chance for success. Both doctors and patients may have trouble saying no if there is "even a small chance it might work."

Under our current medical system patients who want heroic measures usually get them. Increasingly it is being recognized that the pressure to say yes and the difficulty of saying no are too difficult for the individual clinician to deal with alone. Professional standards, hospital policies, and required second opinions are increasingly forcing doctors and patients to constrain this longshot effect.

Thus mistakes in therapeutic decision making often result from doctors' and patients' difficulty with perceptions of probability, evaluation of the utilities of outcomes, and failure to recognize deviations from risk neutrality. Additional errors, as we will see, result from the way the data or pertinent information is conveyed by the physician to the patient. Let us take a look at the problems that occur in the process of uncoerced decision making.

## Uncoerced Decision Making

While overt threats to withhold medical care are easy to recognize and avoid, the goal of conveying pertinent information without coercion is not easy to achieve. Subtle coercion occurs when clinicians present the data in a way that distorts how it is perceived by patients. Doctors may turn the dread effect or the imaginability effect around and use it to increase the patient's fear of the disease or of a particular therapy. The real but small danger of AIDS from blood transfusions, for instance, might be used to deter a patient from surgery. Likewise, the small risk of catastrophic duodenal ulcer perforation might be used to encourage duodenal ulcer surgery.

A very common and difficult-to-avoid process is known as the framing effect. Clinicians may emphasize the five percent probability of death or the 95 percent probability of survival. How the issue is framed by the clinician has a powerful impact on the patient. While it is difficult to totally avoid the framing effect, its impact can be minimized by presenting data both ways. The clinician can first emphasize the probability of death, then the probability of survival. In addition, at times it is helpful to have the patient repeat back his or her understanding of the data. The clinician can then readily recognize whether the patient saw the glass as half full or half empty and can then emphasize the other side of the coin.

The framing effect is not only the result of the words we use to present the data, it is also produced by the tone we employ. Expression of the "facts", stated without pauses or hesitations often convey to the patient professional authority and certainty beyond what we know or intend to convey. In addition, detailed descriptions of the dose and intervals of the treatment often convey a physician's greater familiarity with and confidence in the therapy compared to talking about the treatment in generalities. "We'd like you to agree to take 60mg of adriamycin by intravenous administration every three weeks," carries far more authority and implied certainty than, "we'd like like to give you a trial of adriamycin chemotherapy." The framing effect is difficult for clinicians to eliminate. In fact, physicians who are most adept at developing rapport with patients may be the ones most likely to subtly abuse their ability to convince patients[9].

Having dealt with the differences in perceptions of probability, utility, and risk, and having conveyed the pertinent information in a way that is free of coercion, the doctor and the patient usually will agree. At other times they will at least agree to disagree and will understand where they differ. Occasionally, however, the clinician will have difficulty understanding why the patient refused a therapy or wishes to pursue a particular course of treatment. At these times it is worth reexploring the remaining criteria of informed consent—the capacity to decide.

## Capacity to Decide

Patients initially identified as having the capacity to decide should not be reclassified as not having that capacity simply because we fail to understand their thinking processes or disagree with their choices. At times adult patients' decisions may not seem logical to us, yet they may be based on well-established belief systems, such as those of Christian Scientists. However, if doubts about the patient's capacity to decide are raised, a clinician should know how to begin the difficult process of assessing a patient's capacity to decide.

The ability to understand and communicate choices is obviously impaired when the patient has impaired consciousness. Understanding requires more than consciousness and concentration. Often we use stability of decisions as evidence of understanding. When in doubt, the stability of a patient's decision should be evaluated by repeated questioning over a period of time. The patient who expresses different decisions every few hours often has substantial impairment in capacity to decide.

Patients' ability to rationally manipulate information may be impaired by severe deficits of attention span, intelligence, and memory. Patients' ability to rationally manipulate information can be initially tested by asking the patient to paraphrase in his or her own words what he or she has been told. Of course, this assumes clear communication on the part of the clinician. Patients should also be asked if they understand the purpose of the consent process with such questions as, "What is going to happen if

you sign this form?" The patient's ability to
appreciate the situation and its consequences is
more difficult to assess. However, questions such as,
"What's wrong with you," and "Why are you being
advised to have surgery?" often help identify patients with reduced capacity to decide.

The ability to appreciate the situation and its consequences for their lives may initially be assessed
simply by asking patients "What is most important
to your decision to have (or not have) this procedure?" "Recognizable reasons" for the patient's
choices, such as, "It's too dangerous" or "I want to
get rid of the pain," suggest that the patient has an
adequate capacity to appreciate the situation and its
consequences for their lives[10]. Assessing capacity
to decide may be very difficult, and when doubts are
raised, physicians may require medical and legal
consultation. When patients have (and they usually
do have) the capacity to decide, a method known as
judgment analysis may be helpful. Judgment analysis has been developed to help analyze what is
going on in these types of situations when doctors
have difficulty understanding patients' decisions.
According to Eraker and Politser[11] there are two
common types of impaired judgment that clinicians
need to recognize. Clinicians need to recognize the
existence of impaired judgment when the patient's
current choices are inconsistent with his or her past
behavior or attitudes. The patient who seeks amniocentesis to determine if her fetus has Down's syndrome, but adamantly opposes abortion, may place a
high premium on prognosis or may be displaying inconsistency in her decisions. Inconsistency in decision making is often effectively dealt with by simply
feeding back to the patient the inconsistency. "On
the one hand you seem to want amniocentesis but
you also won't have an abortion if Down's syndrome
is found. Could you help me understand your thinking here?" This type of questioning may help the pa-

tient think through her own decision making process. Patients ultimately have the right to be inconsistent or to choose to have a Down's Syndrome child but the clinician has a responsibility to recognize the problem, confront the patient, and try to connect the patient with their own values.

A second common cause of impaired judgment occurs when the patient's mental state prevents him or her from adequately focusing on the decision. Anxiety and depression are common causes of inattention or misperception. While these conditions usually do not and should not keep a patient from having the capacity to decide, they may prevent patients from hearing, thinking, and judging. When clinicians recognize problems caused by emotional factors, a useful strategy is often to delay the decision and pay attention to the emotional situation. A variety of therapies for anxiety or depression can produce a situation in which patients will be able to focus and utilize their capacity to decide.

The use of judgment analysis also requires that the clinician recognize that how and when information is communicated affects how well patients are able to utilize the information. The patient who has just received a diagnosis of breast cancer is usually not prepared to make decisions on the spot. The reality needs to sink in, and the patient needs time before being able to utilize his or her full facilities.

When patients' decisions don't seem to make sense we need to be sure they have really understood the information. It's not just a matter of repeating the data. It's critical to learn to detect what is blocking a patient from absorbing and dealing with critical data. Often patients can be helped by asking, "What do you think will happen," or "What are you most afraid of?" These questions often elicit the specific fears that keep the patient from hearing all that is said. Patients may not be able to get beyond their fear of pain, vision of being on a respirator, or memory of their family member dying after surgery.

Often we can help patients develop judgments that reflect their own values if we can identify what is going on in their thought processes. For instance, patients often make false associations believing that because they are similar to or close to another person they will react in the same way medically. Their best friend may have gotten an ulcer or become impotent while on a particular medication, and the patient is often sure the same thing will happen to him. Identifying the false association may help us deal with the problem by altering the therapy, providing extra precautions, or explaining to the patient why the situation is different. Even more difficult to deal with is the patient who reverses cause and effect, believing a much needed medication caused a bad outcome. The patient may be thinking, "My mother died within six months of starting high blood pressure medicine. I know it will happen to me too." Patients who fail to recognize their reversal of cause and effect may be among the most difficult to help. They are likely to tune out when presented with additional data. Involving family members who recall how seriously ill their mother was before starting medication or agreeing to start the patient on a very low dose to avoid side effects and gain his or her confidence may help get him or her past the difficult hurdle.

Thus therapeutic decision making involves two separate but closely intertwined processes: the clinician's therapeutic recommendation and the patient's informed consent. Errors in omitting either step are common in medical care. Medical mistakes in therapeutic decision making may be related to differences or distortions in how doctors and patients perceive the probability of the risks and benefits or evaluate the utilities. They may also be due to differences in risk-aversive or risk-seeking attitudes.

In addition to errors resulting from differences in how doctors and patients see the facts, clinicians may contribute to medical mistakes by the way they present the data. Finally, despite pertinent information and uncoerced decision making in a patient who has the capacity to decide, some patients will exhibit barriers to receiving the data. Clinicians must learn to recognize these patients and help them utilize their capacity to decide.

Therapeutic decision making is often hard work. In addition, it never produces a completely objective decision or perfect understanding. Thus it is tempting for patients to throw up their hands and merely tell the doctor to do what he or she thinks is best. However, before concluding that a patient does not want to be involved in the decision-making process, it is necessary for the physician to try. You may be surprised how much the patient does want to participate in the decisions. Fortunately, perfection is not necessary. What is crucial is a process in which the clinician conveys his or her recommendations, including the rationale for treatment, the major benefits and risk expected, and the available alternatives. The physician then needs to respond to the patient's questions. Despite the built-in difficulty in therapeutic decision making, a little time and attention goes a long way toward improving the process.

Good decisions do not guarantee good results, but they do provide a headstart and provide a basis for accepting the less than desired results. Good decisions, however, have little meaning unless they are successfully implemented. Thus, we turn our attention to the next step in the process—execution of therapy.

# 11

# *Execution of Therapy*

No competent clinician would tolerate an error rate of 50 percent or more in identifying disease or in selecting an appropriate therapy. Often competent clinicians, however, achieve less than 50 percent of the potential benefit of the therapy they recommend because patients do not execute what the clinician intended. No area in medicine offers more immediate promise for improving care since obviously if the patient does not take the treatment it's not going to work.

## COMPLIANCE

Many of the mistakes that occur in the execution of therapy rest on misconceptions about compliance with medical care.* Clinicians often believe they

---

*The word compliance itself has been considered by some to reflect the problem. It implies that the clinician is right and all the patient needs to do is implement the treatment without making a decision. The words adherence or failure of execution of treatment may better reflect the philosophy of informed and involved patient decision making. However, since the word compliance is so thoroughly entrenched in medical vocabulary, it will be used here as well.*

**143**

can easily predict which patients will comply. This
common-sense notion has not held up under careful
investigation. Residents at Johns Hopkins, for example, were shown in an investigation to do little better
than chance in predicting patient compliance[12].
Clinicians often believe that patients who are especially anxious about their problems are especially
anxious to comply. However, high levels of anxiety
often interfere with compliance.

Factors that can help in predicting compliance
have also been identified. Past compliance is the
best predictor of future compliance. Knowing your
patient helps. Compliance with one aspect of care is
a good predictor of compliance with other aspects
of care. For example, a patient started on a beta
blocker who develops bradycardia indicating that
they are taking the medication, is probably taking
not only the beta blocker but other medications as
well. Compliance is most likely when symptoms are
present and are immediately relieved by treatment.
For example, an antacid that relieves ulcer symptoms or an antidiarrheal medication that alleviates
intestinal distress is likely to be taken for at least as
long as the symptoms persist. When treatment must
be continued after symptoms are relieved, compliance declines rapidly. A ten-day course of antibiotics for a strep throat or a urinary tract infection has
a high rate of compliance while symptoms are present. The rate for the full course is much lower, however, with many or even most patients failing to
complete the prescription.

Lowest levels of compliance can be expected in
chronic conditions in which symptoms are absent.
Hypertension is the classic example. In this condition, the entire incentive to life-long therapy must be
based on an intellectual knowledge of the benefits
to be gained. The situation is even worse when the
therapy itself induces adverse effects. Thus, it is not
surprising that failure to take medication remains

the greatest single problem in the care of hypertensives. Clinicians who apply these principles can expect to do much better than chance in predicting compliance, although accuracy in predicting compliance will still be far below 100 percent.

A second, common clinical misconception is the belief that patients who understand the pathophysiology of their disease are much more likely to comply. This common-sense proposition has formed the basis of many traditional efforts to inform patients. Patients may be taught the basic pathophysiology of their disease (e.g., diabetes, hypertension, congestive heart failure) in the hope that this knowledge will aid their compliance with threatment. This form of patient education may increase a patient's satisfaction with medical care. Unfortunately, it does far less to increase their compliance. Information is not enough; knowing what to do and what to expect is more important.

In general, behavioral approaches to improved compliance are more useful than patient information approaches aimed at increasing knowledge of a disease's pathophysiology. Specific instructions on what to do, what to look for, and how to follow-up are an important aspect of behavioral education. Continuity of care and ease of access also contribute. Written instructions specifying the timing and dosage of each medication are also of assistance. Positive feedback and reinforcement of patients' efforts are the mainstays of a successful behavioral approach.

A third misconception is that the patient, not the treatment, predicts compliance. Contrary to common belief, there is no convincing evidence to support the idea that compliance is better among women, patients with more formal education, or those from higher socioeconomic classes. These patient characteristics may influence utilization of medical care, but they do not appear to strongly influence compliance with care.

The complexity of the prescription, on the other hand, does have a major influence on compliance. Patients are often prescribed drugs that require complicated scheduling, for example, one drug every six hours, another one hour before meals, another three times a day, and yet another after meals and at bedtime. Any patient would have difficulty complying with such incompatible dosage schedules. The elimination of unnecessary drugs and the simplification of dosage schedules are important measures for increasing compliance. Clarity of instructions is equally important. Patients remember only a small percentage of the verbal instructions physicians give them. Even motivated patients need written instructions if compliance is to be maximized. Writing down nonprescription medications on a prescription form may also increase their legitimacy and subsequent compliance.

Many drugs produce annoying side effects, especially if started at high initial doses. Patients begun on full doses of diuretics often feel "washed out" and may discontinue the drugs or believe they are "allergic" to them. These effects can usually be avoided if low doses are given initially, followed by a gradual increase in dosage. Headaches from initial use of nitrates are so common that they should be expected. Patients should be warned of their occurrence, and, if troublesome, they should use lower initial dosages. Tolerance or adjustment to these effects often requires gradual increase in dosage and a committment by the patient to temporarily endure the initial side effects. Failure to warn patients and support them through the initial period of side effects often leads to discontinuation of useful and safe therapy.

Having prescribed the "right" therapy for the "right" disease and having given the "right" instruction, many clinicians believe that their job is done.

Failure to recognize prescribing pitfalls, however, can lead to the following types of medical mistakes.

## The Complications of Common Sense

Patients using their common sense can get into trouble. Patients' common sense may lead them to stop blood-pressure medication when they feel better or stop birth control pills when they temporarily discontinue sexual relations. Diabetics routinely stop taking insulin when they cannot eat unless they are specifically instructed to check their blood sugar and respond based on a prearranged plan. Common sense may not always make medical sense. Clinicians need to be aware of the difference and specifically inform the patient.

## The Fallacy of Following Orders

Patients often try to follow orders as they understand them. Continuing to take medications in the face of adverse effects can be quite dangerous. The patient who believes that nitroglycerin is prescribed for relief of chest pain may continue to take one after another in the face of a myocardial infarction. Unless specifically instructed to do so, the patient may not recognize the importance of seeking medical care. Similarly, the patient who has been prescribed isoniazid may continue to take the medication, perservering in the face of nausea because that's what they believe the doctor ordered. Patients need to know that they should stop isoniazid when nausea develops or they may turn reversible hepatitis into an irreversible drug-induced hepatitis.

## The Legacy of Leftovers

Patients often self prescribe using their leftover medication on themselves, their friends, or their family. When a full course of antibiotics, for instance, is indicated, patients need to be told to finish the entire course rather than saving a few for future use. Antiinflammatory medications may cause special problems if patients think they are indicated for pain and take them subsequently to relieve gastrointestinal symptoms. Self-treatment is increasingly acceptable and widely practiced in the United States. If self-treatment is to add to the efficiency and effectiveness of medical care and not delay important medical interventions, clinicians must help by anticipating the problems that can develop.

## The Sequelae of Spectacular Results

The tendency to rely on a therapy that has previously given spectacular results can be lethal. For instance, butazolidine for inflamation often produces dramatically successful results when other antiinflamatory drugs have failed. Patients who have once experienced these spectacular results may seek out prolonged treatment with butazolidine despite the hematological danger of long-term therapy. Clinicians are responsible for carefully instructing patients how and when to use all prescribed treatments. Knowing when to stop treatment is as important as knowing when to start.

## When Annoyance Prevents Adherence

Complicated medical regimens are all too common in today's medical practice. Patients often simplify their own regimen, removing inconvenient or bad-tasting drugs or drugs that they believe are producing side effects. Clinicians who fail to simplify patients' treatment and make it compatible with their patients' lifestyles and their physical limitations may contribute to lack of compliance. A patient on a potassium-depleting diuretic, as well as a bad-tasting potassium supplement, often discontinues the potassium if unaware of the dangers. Failure of patients to comply with disagreeable aspects of a treatment regimen can be anticipated and avoided. Patients need to be warned of the disagreeable aspects of therapy and the importance of compliance. If compliance seems unlikely, alternative therapies may be available, including combinations of potassium-depleting and potassium-sparing diuretics that ensure that if a patient takes one drug he or she takes the other as well.

## When the Patient Isn't the End of the Problem

For individual clinicians and individual patients, it is tempting to forget that disease often does not end with the individual and neither should treatment. Neither doctors nor patients are anxious to inform or treat the patient's sexual partners, yet for many sexually transmitted diseases that is an essential part of executing treatment. Without compliance the disease recurs and spreads. Confidentiality must be maintained as much as possible, but for some conditions it is the physician's responsibility to inform. Increasingly, we need to extend beyond the individual patient. For instance, we may need to test family members for genetic disease and perform genetic counseling.

Improved compliance is possible and is likely to improve care. Don't forget, however, that not all noncompliance is bad. Patients who decide not to comply are making judgments about their care.

Sometimes they are right and we have been wrong. Achieving compliance and success in therapy is ultimately grounded on the doctor-patient relationship. In Chapter 13, we will explore the principles that make this relationship a powerful therapeutic agent in its own right.

## BEHAVIOR MODIFICATION

Success in executing therapy involves more than success in getting patients to follow through with taking their medicine. Often changes in longstanding behaviors are required. Failure to engage patients in a process of changing behavior is one of the most common errors made by clinicians. Clinicians usually limit their involvement to warnings to "stop smoking, lose weight, get on the wagon, take your medicine." The advice comes easily to most clinicians who are used to telling other people what to do. It should come as no surprise that once a patient is aware of the risks, the effects of these admonitions are negligible in and of themselves. The aura of authority does occasionally hold sway, and every experienced clinician can proudly recount examples in which his or her orders to change behavior were actually obeyed. However, doctors' orders are not an end in themselves. They are a beginning of a process that requires doctors' roles and patients' roles. Clinicians will fail to achieve results if they are not able to:

Motivate change
Predict who is likely to change
Help maintain change once it has occurred

### Motivating Change

Fear is the traditional motivator used by clinicians to change behavior. The fear of death and disability are high on the list of the most widely used techniques. Fear, however, is frequently ineffective when patients perceive the personal odds of dire consequences as relatively low. In spite of what doctors say, patients think it "can't happen to me." To shore up this belief, patients often cite examples of individuals they know who live to a ripe old age despite, or even because of, X, Y, or Z. In addition, patients often perceive the consequences of loss of life and limb to be so catastrophic that they block out the thoughts. Like nuclear war, the consequences are literally too horrible to contemplate. Finally, the loss to life and limb is rarely immediate. The longer term the risk, the less tangible the reality. In the short term, the only tangible reality may be the suffering required to change behavior.

Faced with the failure of fear, the clinician has other available methods for successfully motivating patients. Instead of using doubtful, dire, and distant complications to motivate, clinicians can be more successful with likely, non-life–threatening, and immediate consequences. Weight loss might be encouraged by immediate social rewards rather than long-term fears of diabetes or heart attacks. The ability to exercise better, wear stylish clothes, keep a job, or please a spouse may be the most successful motivator.

The fact that patients often need tangible evidence of the consequences of their behavior can be used by clinicians in a variety of ways to motivate behavior. Having patients bring out their wedding dress or high school or college yearbook pictures may help to motivate those who have put on far too many pounds over the years.

Motivation often requires peer pressure and peer support. Recognition of this phenomenon has resulted in a proliferation of self-help groups as well as professionally supervised group therapy. Similar types of spurs to motivation can be used by making behavioral changes into a contest utilizing the spirit of competition. Clinicians don't need to run group therapy to use the motivating forces of peer pressure and competition. A husband and wife, for instance, can be encouraged to go on a diet together. Timing can be everything when it comes to motivation. An encouraging pat on the back when the patient is receptive may do more than a verbal hit over the head when the mind is tuned out or turned elsewhere. Presentations with early symptoms secondary to the behavior are frequently the best times for motivating patients. Gastritis or black-out spells in a drinker or bronchitis in a smoker may be turned into early warning signs. These can be presented to the patient as a sign of worse things to come. Identifying the tangible, immediate, and manageable nature of the problem at a relatively early stage can often help encourage change.

## Prognosticating Change

Choosing the right emphasis at the right moment is the key for busy clinicians who know only too well they can't do everything for every patient. Not knowing when and where to put the emphasis reduces the clinician's success, increases frustration, and too often encourages physicians to stop trying. Knowing when and where requires an ability to prognosticate behavioral change. Identifying those factors that indicate a good and a poor prognosis can help clinicians decide when to put in the time themselves, when to call in help, and when to look for makeshift solutions to limit the losses.

Recognition of the danger of the behavior is a necessary prerequisite to behavioral changes. Rarely adequate by itself, without this recognition little change is likely. Patients who claim they don't drink enough to hurt or smoke enough to count are alerting the physician to their lack of readiness for behavioral change. The patient may not be currently receptive to help, so the clinician needs to be on the lookout for when the patient is ready. The patient's own assessment of the prognosis is probably the best one. Those who don't think they can stop rarely do. Unfortunately those who can "take it or leave it" may take it too often. The best solution at this point may be an open door: "It's not easy," or "I'm available to help," or "Come back when you're ready."

The patient's means of dealing with the behavior can be a tipoff to the prognosis. Those who constantly give excuses for why they need to eat or drink are likely to find reasons to continue. Those who have found benefits, sometimes called secondary gains, from their behavior are the least likely to change. If being obese gets them out of social or even sexual expectations, change is not likely.

Finally tests of prognosis can be very useful. Patients can be asked to keep records of their food intake or alcohol consumption. These records not only give an idea of the pattern and intensity of the problem, but failure to deliver can be regarded as a bad prognostic sign.

Bad prognoses should not be equated with writing off either the patient or the problem. The recognition of a difficult problem may signal a need to call for help from the family or the medical system. Alternatively, a bad prognosis may initiate a search for ways to limit the losses. Setting realistic weight-loss or blood-sugar control goals may be half-way measures that reduce the risk when that's what's realistic.

## Implementing and Maintaining Change

Behavioral modification techniques are generally considered the most successful means for a clinician to help a patient one-on-one. These methods rely on the following principles.

1. Behavioral change requires a separation of the desire from the action. This separation is used to put into place barriers between the desire and the action. Sometimes called crutches, the use of these devices may make the difference between success and failure. Waiting five minutes before a cigarette, snack, or drink provides time to decide. Recording all indiscretions before they are committed places the barrier between the patient and the problem.

2. Behavioral change requires changes in old stimulus-response habits. Having a cigarette with coffee, a drink to watch a movie or play cards, or a snack while reading the newspaper creates stimulus-response reactions that are not easily broken. Efforts to identify these situations and remove the individual at least temporarily from the stimulus may be the only way to interrupt habitual responses.

3. Behavioral modification requires positive and immediate reinforcement to be effective. The need for reinforcement can and should be partially accomplished through the words and reactions of the clinician. Progress, however small, should be praised, although good intentions should not. The need for immediate reinforcement requires that patients provide their own rewards. New clothes, a cleaning service to remove the cigarette stains, or other rewards closely linked to the old behavior are ideal. The patient's ability to control the situation and make the choices is key. Family and friends can be of great assistance if they are informed that praise for performance works better than nagging or needling.

4. Focusing on the patient's excuses for drinking, eating, smoking, or any other behavior is often counterproductive. It distracts attention from the problem and encourages the patient to ask for pity rather then help. A sympathetic ear is, of course, an important aspect of a clinician's role, but putting the attention on helping to change the behavior is critical. Helping patients take responsibility is sometimes incorporated into informal or even formal contracts between patients and themselves or patients and clinicians. The rewards and punishments attached to success or failure can be spelled out. These contracts may be part of behavior change designed to stop adverse behavior or part of contracts to ensure compliance. For instance, an agreement that the patient will call if adverse effects occur is coupled with an understanding that the doctor will be available or provide alternative access and do his or her best to minimize side effects.

5. Anticipating the adverse effects and frustrations of behavioral change is helpful in preparing the patient and maintaining motivation. Patients usually do not realize that after stopping smoking a cough can increase due to the increased ability to expectorate sputum. Confronted with an increased cough, patients often regard it as a sign of failure, believing that stopping smoking is just making them feel worse. Patients who do not anticipate the frustrations and commit to seeing them through have a decreased chance of success. Those who diet often lose considerable weight, mostly in the form of water, during the first week or two. This joy of dieting phase is quickly and dependably followed by a frustration phase in which they usually say "I'm doing everything right and I'm not losing weight." Fail-

ure to anticipate this normal biological process often produces patients who are repeatedly unsuccessful in maintaining weight loss.

6. Behavior change requires long-term efforts to maintain the new behavior, reinforce the changes in lifestyle, and detect early the return to old patterns. A high relapse rate should be expected for all difficult-to-change behaviors. Remember that if the behavior had been easy to change it would not have been perpetuated and would not have been taken to the doctor as a problem. The need to expect and detect relapse requires the development of a system. The patient can look for ways to use peer or social pressure to perpetuate the new behavior by finding peers and social groups who support the patient's efforts. Continued, but less frequent, visits to the doctor may help provide the necessary long-term reinforcement. Learning how to deal with the temptation to return to old patterns is essential to long-term success. Anticipating the problems is helpful in dealing with the temptation. Deciding how to handle the offer of a cigarette or a drink at a party is best thought out beforehand. Deciding how to deal with the old drinking buddy who asks the patient out for just a few drinks is critical. Practicing a few good lines may be enough to give the patient the confidence to resist.

Clinicians can efficiently make a major contribution to patients' behavioral changes if they become comfortable with these basic principles. Knowing the limitations of fears and the power of peers is essential to motivation. Appreciating the need for immediate tangible consequences rather than "it can't happen to me" statistics helps to increase motivation. Learning how to prognosticate helps us know when, and when not, to proceed. Those who appreciate the consequences and acknowledge the problem can be more easily helped by the busy practicing clinician. Those whose words and body language fail to acknowledge a problem are usually much more resistant to change.

Successful initial efforts to gain patient compliance and help patients change behavior usually produce a benefit to the patient. However, we can't assume that this will always occur. Thus we are not done with the PESTER process until we have stepped back and reflected on the results as we will discuss in Chapter 12.

# *12*

# *Reflection*

To maximize the benefits of therapy clinicians need to systematically monitor and adjust or change the therapy in light of the patient's response. When therapy is less than optimally successful, the problem may lie with the therapy or with the diagnosis. Before reconsidering either the diagnosis or the therapy, physicians should assume the diagnosis and therapeutic choice were correct and be sure that the patient is actually following the treatment. Failure to follow the therapy, as we have discussed, is far and away the number one cause of therapeutic failure. However, it is not the only cause. When the patient is taking the therapy as prescribed, we must rethink the diagnosis and rethink the therapy to uncover specific causes of failure.

## RETHINKING THE DIAGNOSIS

Therapeutic failure requires that the clinician return to the diagnosis process. Having established that the therapy was actually followed, the first question to ask is whether or not the right diagnosis was made. Infectious diseases, unlike many illnesses, can often be traced to specific, clearly recognizable causes. Even with infectious diseases, however, the laboratory can produce misleading results. Cultures may grow pneumococcus when it is merely colonizing the throat. Diseases requiring small numbers of organisms such as *Giardia* may be entirely missed. The failure of therapy must force one to rethink the disease even when a positive culture is present.

Progression of the disease itself may make therapy more difficult. Vegetations developing from bacterial endocarditis may sequester organisms protecting them from antibiotics. Acidosis, hypoxia, and shock may inhibit the response to antibiotics. Progression of the natural history of diabetes mellitus may alter the insulin requirements in either direction. Progressive disease may necessitate an increased dose, but progressive renal disease or the "honeymoon effect" that occurs early in the course of type I diabetes may actually reduce the need for insulin.

Just as we need to rethink the disease component of a diagnosis, we often need to rethink the cause component. For instance, an underlying cause of the disease may perpetuate the infection. Unrecognized foreign bodies may make cure of infection impossible, or underlying obstruction due to cancer may prevent the clearing of infection. Failure of the infection to clear, when evidence suggests that the right drug is being delivered to the right site with the necessary adjunct therapy, requires the clinician to search for additional underlying causes of the disease.

Failure to respond to an infection may be a function of the infection itself or it may be due to underlying host factors. Immune suppression may be due to another complicating disease. Patients with immune suppression due to cancer, HIV infection, bone marrow suppression, or cancer chemotherapy often present with infections. Therapy must often be simultaneously directed against these underlying causes if maximum potential benefit is to be achieved. In addition the treatment may need to be adjusted to take into account the immune suppression. For instance, in the presence of leukopenia an additional antibiotic may need to be added to otherwise broad spectrum coverage. Rethinking the diagnosis means going back to basics and the most basic principle of all is talking to the patient. As Lipp writes, "The wily consultant in every field knows that the quickest, easiest, surest route to clinical problem solving lies in giving the patient an opportunity to tell you what is going on within.[13]" Often the answer to why the therapy didn't work is misunderstood, forgotten, or denied data that only the patient can provide. Having reconsidered the disease and the cause we must think through several types of problems with the therapy itself.

## RETHINKING THE THERAPY

Initial treatment with drugs such as antibiotics is usually based on the presumed site of infection and knowledge of the likely organisms at that site. Thus it should not be surprising that failures of initial therapy do occur. Some of these can be recognized when unexpected organisms are cultured or antibiotic resistance is demonstrated. The identification of an organism's antibiotic sensitivity often clarifies and redirects therapy. However, in rethinking the therapy it is also important that we look closely at the meaning of the data upon which we have based our decision. For instance, in-vitro laboratory testing for antibiotic sensitivity may differ from the in-vivo situation. Laboratory resistance to isoniazid, for instance, does not correlate well with its actual activity in tuberculosis. With some organisms such as enterococci, disc-susceptibility tests are often mis-

leading. Despite in-vitro sensitivity to single drug
therapy, combination therapy is usually required at
least for infection outside the urinary tract. With
life-threatening diseases such as bacterial endocarditis or sepsis, standard disc sensitivities may not
be sufficient. Dilution methods that assess the sensitivity of the bacteria at varying blood levels of the
drug are helpful in ensuring that standard dosage
schedules are adjusted for the specific organism
and the actual patient.

Occasionally an individual will have two simul-
taneous infections in the same system. Cure of one
infection may allow the other organism to multiply.
Urethritis or cervicitis secondary to gonorrhea may
be accompanied by chlamydia. Cure of the gonorrhea
may allow the chlamydia to multiply, producing the
clinical syndrome of post-gonococcal urethritis,
which requires a course of a tetracycline for cure.
The Centers for Disease Control recommend treatment for chlamydia whenever gonorrhea is identified.

In addition to rethinking the therapy by reevaluat-
ing the meaning of the data used to reach an initial
therapeutic decision, it is important to ask why the
therapy may not be working.

Grahame-Smith and Aronson[14] have identified
four processes that occur in drug therapy. The components of these processes can be used to identify
problems that can occur in achieving successful
therapy, even those that do not utilize drugs. The
processes and questions to ask include:

The pharmaceutical process—is the therapy getting
    to the patient?
The pharmacokinetic process—is the therapy get-
    ting to its site action?
The pharmacodynamic process—is the therapy pro-
    ducing the required biological effects?
The therapeutic process—is the biological effect
    being translated into a therapeutic effect?

## Is the Treatment Getting to the Patient?

Patients may be 'taking' their treatments, yet fail to be taking them properly. Specific questioning may be necessary to recognize, for instance, that bronchodilator inhalants are being used improperly, or that tetracycline is being combined with antacids thereby preventing absorption. Mechanical treatments such as physical therapy, exercise, or a prothesis are particularly likely to be used incorrectly, thereby dramatically reducing their effectiveness.

Even if the patient is taking the treatment properly the treatment may not be bioavailable. Drugs given intervenously all enter the systemic circulation and are considered 100 percent bioavailable. Drugs that require gastrointestinal absorption, however, may not reach the systemic circulation. Before entering the systemic circulation, oral forms of administration must pass several hurdles. Drugs must be delivered in a form that the body can absorb, this is known as pharmaceutical availability. In addition, gastrointestinal absorption must occur and the drug must survive the "first-pass" effect of liver metabolism as it enters the liver's portal circulation. All these barriers may influence the quantity of drug reaching the systemic circulation.

Food and Drug Administration (FDA) approved manufacturing standards are designed to ensure approximately equal pharmaceutical availability of different formulations of the same drug. Recent experience, however, has demonstrated that FDA approved procedures are not always followed. Small differences in serum levels can have large therapeutic consequences. With such drugs as digoxin, warfarin, and anticonvulsant medications physicians need to be especially alert to the potential for differences between different pharmaceutical preparations.

The use of multiple drugs and solutions requires the physician to consider the presence of drug incompatibilities. Antibiotics may be incompatible chemically or physically with IV solutions or other drugs. The activity of gentamicin, for instance, can be reduced when it is mixed with carbenicillin and other penicillins. Amphotericin B may precipitate in saline. Many antibiotics are incompatible with other drugs and should be administered alone. Clinicians are not expected to know all of the possible incompatibilities, but the patient's failure to respond to seemingly appropriate therapy should raise the issue of incompatibility.

Problems with gastrointestinal absorption may result from reduced motility in conditions such as diabetic gastric atony and intestinal ileus, or from bowel wall edema in congestive heart failure. Inadequate or undependable gastrointestinal absorption is such a frequent problem that use of parenteral treatments should be considered for seriously ill patients.

The liver's ability to protect the systemic circulation from many poisons that enter the GI tract also results in rapid metabolism and potentially ineffective therapy with medications that undergo extensive first-pass metabolism, such as propranolol and orally administered nitrates.

Thus whenever the patient is taking the treatment but it is not working the first questions to ask are, "Is the patient taking the treatment properly and is the therapy bioavailable?"

## Is the Treatment Getting to Its Site of Action?

To achieve its intended effect a therapy must adequately reach its site of action. For drug treatments, adequate blood levels are required as well as adequate penetration to the site of action. Adequate blood levels may not occur because of variations in protein binding, renal excretion, and metabolism. For a select number of drugs, monitoring of blood levels can be helpful. Monitoring of serum levels of theophylline, phenytoin, and quinidine may help to ensure therapeutic effectiveness.

Drug interactions are becoming recognized as a major source of ineffective treatment in addition to their effects on safety. Patients taking great numbers of drugs are especially prone to these problems. It is impossible to memorize the rapidly growing list of drug interactions, but a high level of suspicion and frequent efforts to look it up can keep this from becoming an unnecessary cause of therapeutic failure.

Adequate blood levels may not be sufficient when barriers exist to penetration of the drug to the site of action. In shock the circulation may be inadequate for the drug to reach the target organ. Many drugs fail to cross the blood-brain barrier when inflammation subsides. In addition, penetration of the prostate and walled off abscesses may prevent adequate medical treatment. Clinicians must be alert to the need to consider switching drugs or substituting surgery.

Treatments other than drugs may also have problems getting to the site of action. Externally applied heat, for instance, may not penetrate through fat to reach the underlying muscle. Thus when asking whether the treatment is getting to the site of action, clinicians need to consider whether adequate levels of therapy have been maintained and whether the therapy is penetrating to the site of action.

## Is the Treatment Producing the Required Biological Effect?

Even at therapeutic levels treatments may fail to produce their intended biological effects. Failure may occur because drugs may induce their own effects that counter their primary action. Alternatively a variety of mechanisms may induce tolerance to the effect, thus reducing the biological consequences of the treatment. Drugs such as carbamazepine and phenobarbital may induce their own hepatic metabolism. Protective homeostatic mechanisms may reduce drug effectiveness. Antihypertensive medications such as methyldopa and clonidine when used alone may lose effectiveness over time as they induce fluid retention and the blood pressure slowly rises.

Tolerance is said to be occurring when prior exposure results in biological modification that reduces the effectiveness of subsequent doses. Tolerance is not limited to narcotics and other centrally acting depressants. Nitrates given as continuous absorption preparations have been shown to lose effectiveness when administered on a 24 hour per day basis. Effectiveness, however, can be maintained when nitrate patches are removed at night.

## Has the Biological Effect Been Translated into a Therapeutic Effect?

Even when treatments produce their intended biological effect the patient may not benefit adequately. The disease may be simply too severe for the treatment to work. Adult onset diabetes mellitus may not adequately respond to oral hypoglycemic agents and insulin may need to be substituted. Similarly nonsteroidal antiinflammation treatment for rheumatoid arthritis may not produce an adequate response. Thus, the clinician faced with a biological effect but inadequate therapy needs to ask: Are there acceptable alternatives? At times the question becomes, can we settle for a partial response?

The search for the causes of therapeutic failure has led us to retrace the steps in the diagnostic process as well as the therapeutic process. This retracing is important to recognize since it reminds us that medical decision making is not a linear process. Therapeutic decision making is a dynamic process. What is appropriate therapy at the onset may become inappropriate as the patient fails to respond. The response must be continually reassessed if optimal results are to be obtained. Recognizing the uncertainty of even appropriate therapy should lead clinicians to systematically and routinely search for what went wrong.

We have now taken a step-by-step look at the PESTER process of therapeutic decision making including Prognosis, Effectiveness, Safety, Therapy, Execution, and Reflection. We have outlined what needs to be accomplished in each of these components, pointed out errors that occur in each step, and suggested ways to prevent or identify early some of these errors of implementation. Now let us turn to the final part of the book and take a look at what else matters.

## REFERENCES

1. Feinstein AR. An additional basic science for clinical medicine I. The constraining fundamental paradigms. *Ann Intern Med* 99:393–97, 1983.

2. Thomas L. *The Youngest Science: Notes of a Medicine-Watcher*. Toronto: Bantam, 1983.

3. Forster LE, Lynn J. The use of physiologic measures and demographic variables to predict longevity among inpatient hospice applicants. *Am J Hospice Care* 6:31–34, 1989.

4. Strauss MB, (Ed.) *Familiar Medical Quotations*. Boston: Little, Brown, 1968.

5. Lambert EC. *Modern Medical Mistakes*.

Bloomington: Indiana University Press, 1978. P. 11.

6. Steel K. Latrogenic illness on a general medical service at a university hospital. *N Engl J Med* 304:638–42, 1981.

7. President's commission for the study of ethical problems in medicine and biomedical and behavior research. *Making Health Care Decisions*. Washington, D.C.: U.S. Government Printing Office, 1982. P. 57–8.

8. Mazur DJ. Why the goals of informed consent are not realized. *J Gen Intern Med* 3:370–380, 1988.

9. Arnold R, Povar G, and Howell J. The humanities, humanistic behaviors and the humane physician: A cautionary note. *Ann Intern Med* 106(2):313–18, 1987.

10. Applebaum PS, Grisso T. Assessing patients' capacities to consent to treatment. *N Engl J Med* 319:1635–8, 1988.

11. Eraker SA, Politer P. How decisions are reached: Physician and patient. *Ann Intern Med* 97:262–268, 1982.

12. Haynes BR, Taylor DW, and Sackett DC (Eds.) *Compliance in Healthcare*. Baltimore: Johns Hopkins University Press, 1979. P. 46–62.

13. Lipp MR. Respectful Treatment: A Practical Handbook of Patient Care (2nd ed.). New York: Elsevier, 1986.

14. Grahame-Smith OG, Aronson JK. *Oxford Textbook of Clinical Pharmacology and Drug Therapy*. Oxford: Oxford University Press, 1984.

# III

## *What Else Matters*

# 13

# *Building Toward TRUST*

Throughout the history of medicine trust has formed the basis of the doctor-patient relationship. Until recently, however, trust meant the delegation of the authority for decision making to the doctor. Doctors, acting in patients' "best interests" would do what they thought was best. Keeping patients in the dark was regarded as more efficient than involving patients in a complex process. In addition it was thought to increase the effectiveness of therapy by removing doubt or uncertainty. The patient trusted the doctor, and the doctor was entrusted with the patient's care. The traditional doctor-patient relationship was based on therapeutic blind trust, denial of uncertainty, and withholding of unpleasant truths. Today doctor-patient relationships are still central to the success of medical care. However, these relationships need to be based on therapeutic relationships, uncertainty sharing, and truth. We may combine these three essential features of the modern doctor-patient relationship and remember them by using the mnemonic TRUST.

Therapeutic
Relationship
Uncertainty
Sharing
Truth

## THERAPEUTIC RELATIONSHIP

Trust remains central to the therapeutic effects of
doctor-patient relations. However, the meaning of the
words has changed. In the *Silent World of Doctor
and Patient*, Katz writes that, "Trust based on blind
faith . . . must be distinguished from trust that is
earned[1]."

The relationship between doctor and patient goes
beyond an exchange of data, it can actually become
part of the therapy. Physicians have long recognized
the power of the therapeutic relationship incorporated in the placebo effect. The traditional use of
placebos has meant presenting biologically inert
substances as biologically active. Controlled clinical
trials that use placebos as a justified form of patient
deception have established beyond a reasonable
doubt that placebos work.

In his review of the placebo effect, Brody[2] has
written that "although placebos are commonly
thought of primarily as pain relievers, virtually all
potentially reversible symptoms and diseases that
have been investigated in double-blind studies show
some response to placebo—including diabetes, angina and malignant neoplasms." Blind faith was
once believed to be a prerequisite for eliciting the
placebo effect. Yet as Brody writes, it is possible
through a therapeutic relationship to elicit "a placebo effect without the placebo[2]." To recognize the
scientific basis of the placebo effect we need to integrate it into the therapeutic relationship in a way
that complements the science and legitimatizes the
art of medicine.

While there are many methods that work for many different doctors the following four basic components are usually part of a successful therapeutic relationship. They can be summarized and remembered using the mnemonic SURE.

**S**upport
**U**nderstanding
**R**espect
**E**mpathy

## Support

Support is a basic prerequisite of the therapeutic relationship. It implies that the doctor intends to be of help. Often this is assumed and the doctor needs to do no more. At times, however, it is not obvious to the patient that the doctor is on his or her side. The disability exam, the company doctor, the physician who is paid more to do less may put all physicians in the position of needing to convince the patient that they intend to give support. Support is often demonstrated by steps that legitimize a patient's problem. Letting the patient know that his or her feelings are a normal or even healthy reaction, supporting reasonable leave requests, or promptly filling out needed insurance papers may also facilitate the feeling of support. Providing support can be conveyed directly by such expressions as, "I would like to help you get to the bottom of this problem," or "Let's see what we can both do to help you stop smoking."

Providing support does not mean that the physician needs to take on all the responsibility for medical care or emotional support. Often the critical role is mobilizing the resources of the medical system, the family, and the community. Perhaps the most important resources, however, are those of the patients themselves. This type of support often requires patients to realize that the doctor is there to help them get better, not make them get better. Thus, part of the process of support is to bolster the role of the patient in the therapeutic process.

Even in surgery, where the physician seems ultimately in control, Selzer writes, "The surgeon is the mere instrument which the patient takes to his hand to heal himself[3]." In surgery the patient's willingness to limit narcotics, ambulate despite pain, and actively participate in treatment often requires the patient's determination to recover. The power of the placebo effect to promote self healing often requires willingness by the patient to take on the responsibility and ultimately the credit for the success of treatment. A successful outcome is often heralded by the patient's acceptance of the need for action and change and claiming it as his or her own idea.

## Understanding

Understanding implies that the patient feels that he or she has been heard, that the problem has registered in the doctor's consciousness, and that the doctor is thinking about the problem. A verbal or nonverbal "I hear you, I understand what you're saying to me" can aid understanding. Understanding is often conveyed by the physician's nonverbal communication such as eye contact, nodding your head, or semi-verbal expressions of interest such as "uh-huh." The clinician's tone and intonation may convey attention and understanding or remoteness and disinterest. Clinicians can consciously convey interest and understanding by using such expressions as "please go on," and "tell me more," or by repeating the patient's previous words, demonstrating that you have been listening. According to Quill, physicians need to recognize when an understanding does not exist and identify the barriers. Often physicians can identify these barriers because the patient is giving them contradictory information with words or with words plus nonverbal messages. At other times barriers can be recognized because the physician feels uncomfortable or the patient puts up resistance. For instance, a patient may resist answering questions saying he or she is tired of having people "poking into" his or her personal life. Noncompliance and treatment failures may be the only sign that barriers to understanding exist. When these barriers do not easily fall, Quill suggests saying, "I'm sensing you are unhappy with the direction I am proposing but I'm not sure why. Perhaps you could help me understand what is going on[4]." Patients will often convey their anxiety to physicians by the use of humor. Comments like "I don't think I'll be trying out for the Olympics now," or "This should keep me off the street" require a response from the doctor. Often a smile is all that is necessary, or a simple "I know how you feel" can go a long way toward conveying understanding.

## Respect

Respect for patients implies a recognition of the importance of the patients as individuals and the importance of their problems. Respect goes beyond acknowledging that they have been heard and reflects that their problems matter. Recognition of what the patient is going through is often crucial to achieving a sense of respect. The doctor needs to say in effect, "I appreciate why you're frustrated with your slow recovery, your long waits to be seen, your worsening symptoms."

Respect is often conveyed by learning enough about a patient's personal and professional life to be able to view him or her as a person, not only as a patient. Taking the time to be aware of patients' ac-

complishments and attitudes is in itself a sign of respect. Often all that is necessary is active attention.
Simple things like remembering patients' names,
and calling them by their last names unless you are
particularly familiar are important. Nonverbal communication often helps reinforce or destroy respect.
Looking patients in the eyes and sitting at their level
can convey respect. Continuous interruptions or
medical discussions in the patient's presence that
exclude the patient can destroy respect. Appropriate
praise can gain respect, for instance, letting patients
know that their efforts to comply are appreciated
goes a long way. Letting them know that the old x
ray they obtained was very helpful is important positive feedback that conveys respect. On the other
hand, one of the most dangerous and destructive
practices is the use of belittling remarks. Patients
who overhear physicians making fun of them are
not likely to forgive or forget. Whether correctly or
incorrectly interpreted, overheard remarks are the
making of malpractice suits.

## Empathy

Empathy is a key ingredient in the doctor-patient relationship. It requires doctors to be able to put themselves in patients' situations and view the world
through patients' eyes. Empathy can often be conveyed merely by identifying with the patient's experience
and then labeling the resulting emotion: "It sounds
like you've been through a tough time, it must have
made you angry," or "It sounds like people have let
you down, you must have been disappointed."
    Compassion is the emotion we experience and con-
vey when we exhibit empathy. Compassion, derived
from latin roots, means to suffer with or to experience with. Suffering with patients starts by being
there, often saying nothing, waiting for the patient to

speak. Taking the time and letting the patient know you'll be back and that you will follow-up.

Compassion requires physicians to allow patients to tell and sometimes retell their story and to allow patients to deal with the consequences of their disease and its meaning to their lives. Empathy can be and often is accomplished using the traditional laying on of hands, the reaching out and touching patients literally and emotionally. As Rynearson has written, "Physicians need to be in actual touch with patients. Increasingly technology in medicine is pushing the physician away from the patient. If the physician allows machinery to be interposed between him and the patient, he will be in danger of forfeiting powerful healing influences[5]."

Once formed, a therapeutic relationship is a central part of the delivery of medical care. As Balint wrote in his classic study of doctor-patient relationships, "... by far the most frequently used drug ... was the doctor himself ...[6]." Confirming this from the patient's point of view Cousins wrote, "In this sense the doctor himself is the most powerful placebo of all[7]."

The therapeutic relationship is not only curative in its own right, it also augments and facilitates other therapies. For instance, compliance often depends on the development of a therapeutic relationship. Similarly, a productive doctor-patient relationship is often the key to motivating patients to engage in the difficult process of behavior change. Thus, beyond its inherent value, the doctor-patient relationship is often a prerequisite to, and a sustaining force behind, the success of other therapies.

Clinicians are usually fortunate since patients seeking medical care usually expect to form a therapeutic relationship with their physician aimed at dealing with their presenting problems. However, this is not always the case. It is important for clinicians to recognize signs and symptoms of:

Patients who do not seek a therapeutic relationship.
Patients who seek to utilize the doctor-patient relationship to fulfill other agendas.
Patients with whom physicians find it difficult to form a therapeutic relationship.
Situations where even an effective doctor-patient relationship hinders the recognition of new problems.

## Patients Who Do Not Seek a Therapeutic Relationship

In today's medical environment, patients may come to the doctor skeptical of the willingness or ability of the doctor to help. These patients are usually not initially prepared to develop a therapeutic relationship. Medical students have long recognized that patients often regard their interaction as a mandatory prerequisite to receiving care. This same skepticism may be sensed by primary-care clinicians, who the patient may view as "gatekeepers", keeping them from receiving needed services. The request to see a specialist even before completing their history may be the not-too-subtle tip-off that the patient is not seeking a therapeutic relationship. At times patients may signal their attitudes by overt warnings such as, "I don't like coming to doctors" or "Medicine never does much good", or even "I don't have much faith in medicine."

Recognition of patients who are skeptical of doctors and medicine is usually quite simple. The tendency to react negatively or defensively, however, may be harder to avoid. Yet it is important to recognize these patients and avoid trying to convince them by your words. They are likely to be much more receptive to what you do than what you say. Letting patients know they've been heard can be very helpful in this and many areas of potential doctor-patient conflicts. Sometimes a direct "I hear you," or "I'll be giving you my recommendation. The decisions, of course, are yours," can turn the corner and let the patient relax.

## Using the Doctor-Patient Relationship to Fulfill Other Agendas

Patients who seek to utilize the doctor-patient relationship to fulfill other agendas may be more difficult to recognize. These patients, unlike those who are skeptical of medical care, often appear cooperative, appreciative, and even trusting. In fact, the patient who goes overboard with his or her praise is a prime candidate to destroy the therapeutic relationship. According to Hahn and colleagues, there are two basic types of situations where patients often seek a "dysfunctional compensatory alliance." One such situation occurs "wherever patients in words and actions, attempt to engage the clinician in an alliance and to take his or her 'side' against other family members: 'Tell my wife that I am . . .' or 'It's my husband's fault that I'm depressed . . .'[8]."

In this form of dysfunctional relationship the clinician becomes a weapon for the patient to use in a struggle with family members or other important persons. The doctor may then be asked to intervene on the patient's behalf to take the patient's side in an ongoing struggle. These types of requests to get in the middle should be seen as warning signs that the therapeutic relationship may be being used to serve other patient agendas. Having recognized the potential for this type of dysfunctional relationship, it is often necessary to bring in the other individual, usually in the same room at the same time with the patient. Without making accusations, it is important that everyone hear your conclusions and recommendations at the same time in the same way or they may be distorted in the translation.

A second type of situation in which the doctor-patient relationship may become dysfunctional rather than therapeutic occurs when a patient's disease or his behavior results in secondary gain. Secondary gain means that the patient gains something from the symptoms or illness, and the patient is thus very resistant to giving up his or her symptoms. The gain may be attention, reduced responsibilities, or special privileges attached to being sick. Thus in the words of Hahn and colleagues the patient has a "need to be sick" and uses the doctor-patient relationship to gain an "official seal of approval[8]. "We may give our seal of approval by giving the patient a label called a disease, giving medications, recommending pleasurable activities, or restricting unpleasurable ones. This can be a particularly difficult situation for clinicians who often feel the desire or need to bend-over-backward to support the patient in dealing with the outside world. It may be necessary to say in effect, "I'll be as supportive as I can, but you know I have to be able to defend what I say." Thus, it is important to recognize patients who utilize the doctor-patient relationship for secondary gain, for they can be easily confused with patients who seek a truly therapeutic relationship.

Both of these types of dysfunctional relationships are characterized by little change in patient behavior over time and often a sense of frustration and even anger and helplessness on the part of the clinician. Doctors must be alert to the situation in which the doctor-patient relationship is being used to fulfill other agendas, or clinicians will feel used and abused and patients will not benefit.

A final type of patient who does not seek a therapeutic relationship is the rare patient who has been called "suit prone." In recent years malpractice suits have grown in frequency and financial impact to the point that most doctors will get sued at some time during their careers. Thus most doctors now legitimately fear the dangers to their reputation, the personal emotional turmoil, and the enormous consumption of their limited time. Lawyers tell physicians that the best defense in a malpractice suit is good documentation, formal informed consent, and early detection of problems, followed by a prompt response to medical mistakes. Serious errors in diagnosis or therapy may result in a lawsuit even when a good doctor-patient relationship is present, but it is important to recognize that most malpractice suits are really a symptom of the breakdown of the doctor-patient relationship. The best malpractice prevention often requires concentration on the doctor-patient relationship. Malpractice prevention by attention to the doctor-patient relationship is important for all patients.

Despite their rarity, it is important for clinicians to be able to recognize patients who are prone to lawsuit. This can be done without becoming obsessed by the possibility of a malpractice suit. These patients may occasionally be recognized by their history of previous multiple malpractice suits. Unfortunately, patients who have sued before are more likely to sue again. In addition, patients with unrealistic expectations about what can be accomplished medically are also prone to lawsuit when disappointment sets in. Patients who flatter us into thinking we can do the impossible or nearly impossible should also put us on guard rather than in the clouds. There are no easy answers for dealing with these patients. Here, however, the lawyer's frequent advice to doctors should be followed: document, document, document, and do it legibly.

## Patients Physicians Find Difficult

There are certain types of patients who pose difficulties when we try to form a therapeutic

relationship. These are often patients we don't care
for because of their personality characteristics. As
physicians it is important to be able to care for
patients one doesn't like. Patient types that
physicians often find difficult according to Groves[9]
include entitled demanders, dependent clingers, and
manipulative help rejectors. Entitled demanders
make unreasonable demands sound legitimate.
Dependent clingers utilize medical services to the
point where they produce irritation and annoyance.
Manipulative help rejectors frustrate and often
annoy physicians by repeatedly reporting treatment
failures. It is important to remember, however, that
the patients whom physicians find difficult also
include patients with diagnosable and treatable
diseases who present with atypical symptoms.
Despite the fact that difficult patients are not the
rule they may have a disproportionate effect on
physicians who don't know how to handle the
situation. Psychiatrists have long recognized that
their reactions to a patient often give them insight
into how the patient is received by others. The
demanding, dependent, or manipulative patient who
elicits negative feelings in us usually produces
negative responses in others as well.

Nesheim suggests paying attention to your reactions, "Your first awareness that something is wrong
here is critical . . . Take special note of those patients whose phone messages evoke despair and
whose clinical visits cloud an entire afternoon." The
appreciation that others must react the same way
helps clinicians establish the necessary emotional
distance to objectively deal with the patient effectively. Performing a second differential diagnosis is
the next step. According to Nesheim this informal
differential "should include personality considerations as well as the more formal diagnostic categories of psychiatric disease. Is the patient demanding
too much? Challenging your competence or authori-

ty in your area of expertise? Is a covert but diagnosable psychiatric disorder present—a masked depression presenting as physical complaints, a delusional state with a somatic presentation and underlying disordered thinking, or perhaps occult chemical dependency[10]?"

What should be done for these difficult patients who do not have an identifiable medical or psychiatric diagnosis? Accepting the symptoms as real without identifying a disease is key. Identifying a disease usually makes life difficult later when the patient is convinced he or she has disease X. Alpert and Wittenberg offer suggestions for dealing with entitled demanders, dependent clingers, and manipulative help rejectors. For entitled demanders they suggest, "the physician must recognize and explain to the patient that he or she is entitled to good medical care but not necessarily to his or her particular requests." Presenting options but drawing the line as well may help to deal with the situation. For dependent clingers they recommend regular time-limited scheduled appointments that don't require symptoms to justify the appointment. For manipulative help rejecters they write, ". . . the best plan may be to acknowledge the failure of treatment, share the pessimism, and emphasize the doctor-patient relationship rather than the success of a given program with its implied termination of the relationship[11]."

## Effective Relationships May Hinder Recognition of New Problems

Finally, we need to recognize that the closeness of the doctor-patient relationship may make it difficult for us to step back and see what's really happening. The closeness and trust inherent in the doctor-patient relationship may prevent us from recognizing the patient who is abusing drugs, becoming addicted to treatment, or seeing other doctors to obtain conflicting therapies. Thus it is often helpful to have a colleague take a look at patients you have been following. This new perspective will often provide insights that would be difficult for you to see.

Therapeutic relationships are a fundamental goal of the doctor-patient relationship. Providing support, understanding, respect, and empathy are the goals that allow the physician to achieve the placebo effect without the placebo. However, not all patients seek a therapeutic relationship. Patients may use the doctor-patient relationship to form dysfunctional alliances, and a few patients will be prone to lawsuit. It is important to recognize and be prepared to deal with patients we do not like. At times the closeness of the doctor-patient relationship makes it difficult for clinicians to step back and see what is really going on. The importance of doctor-patient relationships cannot be overemphasized. The ability to obtain and sustain therapeutic relationships is often what patients view as the most important characteristic they look for in a doctor.

## UNCERTAINTY SHARING

As Osler wrote over a half century ago, "Medicine is a science of uncertainty and an art of probability.[12]" Every probability of being right implies a probability of being wrong. Increasingly, today's clinicians are coming to realize that uncertainty and doubt are an intrinsic part of the practice of medicine. Uncertainty can be measured, reduced, and characterized, but it can't be eliminated. Thus, as an old Chinese proverb says, "To be uncertain is uncomfortable; to be certain is ridiculous." It is increasingly important that physicians learn to acknowledge the existence of uncertainty and learn to live with it. A basic

approach to living with uncertainty is learning to
share it comfortably with patients.

In an era when doctors are expected to share
decision making through informed consent, clinicians
also need to learn to share the accompanying
uncertainty. As Gutheil and colleagues have written,
"The real clinical opportunity offered by informed
consent is that of transforming uncertainty from a
threat to the doctor-patient alliance into the very basis
on which an alliance can be formed[13]." This alliance,
they feel, not only serves the patient's interest, but
provides the clinician with his or her best protection
against suit. Patients who feel that they have made the
decision to have surgery or accept the dangers of
medication are more likely to view any consequences
as known risks rather than negligence.

Uncertainty sharing is not an easily learned art.
Patients may resist sharing uncertainty, perhaps
hoping to place both the decision making and the
responsibility for the outcome in the hands of the
clinician. Doctors, too, may have trouble sharing uncertainty. They may choose the traditional route of
denying uncertainty and acting as the unquestioned
authority. Alternatively, they may be overwhelmed
by the uncertainty and refuse to make clear-cut recommendations. The pendulum has swung too far
when the doctor in effect says to the patient, "the
choice is yours; I'm not responsible."

Uncertainty is one of the unpleasant facts of life.
Neither doctors nor patients relish the idea of having
to live with and share uncertainty. Thus doctors
may turn to counterproductive means of dealing
with uncertainty, which often constitute medical
mistakes, including:


Excessive testing
Superimposing certainty

## Excessive Testing

Physicians are tempted to treat their own uncertainty and insecurity by ordering tests. Tests are ordered to appropriately reduce uncertainty, then further testing is done to reduce the uncertainty still more. Since it is never possible to be certain, it is always possible to justify testing to reduce the uncertainty. The tendency to equate medicine with detective work leads to many misplaced priorities. The tendency to leave no stone unturned, to tie up all the loose ends, to believe that time is of the essence, belongs more appropriately in the solving of a murder mystery than in medical diagnosis and treatment.

## Superimposing Certainty

Faced with uncertainty, it is tempting for individual physicians and the medical profession to gloss over the inherent uncertainty by superimposing an artificial certainty. As a profession we often create diagnostic categories and therapeutic protocols that proclaim what a condition should be called, what a symptom should be called, or how a symptom should be treated if there is no clear answer. At times this is a helpful approach if it superimposes a reasonable course of action, such as: "It's better to overtreat syphilis if we don't know how long it's been present," or "It's better to hospitalize a patient with chest pain if we can't exclude unstable angina."

At other times superimposing certainty can lead doctors and patients astray. Classifying high blood pressure as essential hypertension, pancreatitis as idiopathic, or infection as cryptogenic are deceiving ways of hiding our own uncertainty about the cause of the disease. The creation of diagnoses of exclusion that do not themselves have position criteria for diagnosis may create "wastebasket" categories. These diagnostic categories may produce a label that has little meaning because it does not provide a reliable prognosis or treatment. Disease categories like viral infection or irritable bowel disease may hide more than they reveal, by providing both patients and doctors with unwarranted certainty.

How can a physician deal with uncertainty without relying on excessive testing or superimposed certainty? Hilfiker suggests some possible ways. "The physician can provide useful information and support to the patient 'It doesn't seem serious', 'It will pass on its own', or 'It's normal to experience this' . . .[14]." The physician is dealing with the patient's concerns and providing a prognosis rather than a precise diagnosis. Patients are often willing to forego the formalities of a diagnostic evaluation if they can feel confidence in the future. Often, of course, a physician cannot truthfully offer such an optimistic outlook.

Thus in many situations the key is for the physician to recognize that uncertainty is inevitable and not allow it to paralyze necessary action. If we waited for certainty, we'd never cross the street. The inevitability of uncertainty and subsequent error, however, means physicians need to build safety nets into their practices. Close follow-up, such as calling patients back or seeing them the next day, may be the best way to reduce everyone's anxiety. Calling a diagnosis tentative or provisional forces the physician to keep his or her door open. Labeling problems as chest pain or headache of unknown etiology forces physicians to deal with the diagnosis again later. Keeping symptoms separated on the problem list rather than prematurely combining them into a diagnosis keeps the mind open.

In addition, physicians need to deal with the inevitability of error in the medical system in which they work. As Lipp has written:

The rule is: 'The system will screw up. Lab results will be lost. The patient's appointment for cardiac catheterization will get postponed interminably...' Recognize that system failures are inevitable everywhere, not unique to your particular setting. Don't feel a failure or that you work in a lousy place when bad things happen. Just do the best you can... Enlist the patient's assistance. 'If we screw up and you don't hear from us, please call to jog my memory.' Have some system for maintaining continuity where it is needed despite system failures[15].

Uncertainty sharing is not the same as anxiety sharing. Patients may be reassured by a physician's calm, thoughtful, compassionate manner even while their words convey probabilities and uncertainties. As Johnson and colleagues have written, "If the physician is calm, reassuring, empathetic and appears untroubled in the face of uncertainty, patient satisfaction may not be diminished. If the patient feels that the physician is in control, is concerned, and has the optimal care of the patient as the highest priority, dissatisfaction may not occur[16]." Ironically, the sharing of responsibility and uncertainty can be enhanced by empathizing with rather than confronting the patient's unrealistic search for certainty. As Gutheil and colleagues write, "Paradoxically, the best way... is to empathize with the patient's wish for certainty and with its specific manifestations as understandable reactions to a difficult and painful situation... 'I wish I could give you a medication that was sure to have only positive effects' and 'There is just no guarantee you'll live through this — I wish there were,'... invites the patient to exchange idealization for identification.... by the shared acknowledgement of clinical uncertainty and of the fantasies used to deny it[13]."

What do today's clinicians have to take the place of the certainty of another era? We still have one key tool that can be an essential support for patients who are sharing in the uncertainty. We can be with the patient. "I'll be with you every step of the way," writes Gutheil and colleagues, implies the "promise of a continuing relationship, even if there is a tragic outcome. When this promise is fulfilled, the patient is less likely to feel a need to force the physician to share the experience of the misfortune by means of a malpractice suit[13]." Conversely, the doctor who isn't there when the patient expects his or her presence is open to disappointment, hostility, and worse. Nothing is more undermining to the doctor-patient relationship than dashed expectations. Thus, we are led to the final issue of our modern doctor-patient relationship, that of truth.

## TRUTH

In everyday life self denial, social denial, and social inhibitions limit and direct what is acknowledged and what is communicated. Despite the social conventions favoring only limited truth telling, medicine is a forum in which the patient's most intimate secrets are legitimately discussed. As Sokas has said, "Doctors can expect honest answers to questions which even the patient's mother is not allowed to ask[17]." We have already discussed how self denial and social denial affects the clinician's ability to accurately obtain the facts as part of the patient's history. Patients often have even greater difficulty telling themselves the truth about how they feel or why they act the way they do. Problems in truth telling may occur because:

Patients have trouble telling doctors the truth.
Doctors have trouble telling patients the truth.
Doctors have trouble telling themselves the truth.

## Patients Telling Doctors the Truth

The truth telling permitted by the doctor-patient relationship grants doctors the privilege of helping patients acknowledge their true feelings and true motives. Often clinicians become alert to patients' denials by an incongruity between the patients' words, their effect, and/or their body language. When incongruity between a patient's demeanor and words are apparent, valuable insight is often gained by pointing out the incongruity. This is best done by feeding back to the patient what is observed. This can be done without insulting the patient by such expressions as, "you sound angry," "you seem tense," or "you look depressed." This reflecting back to the patient what the physician observes allows the patient the opportunity to reflect on his or her own emotions.

More specifically, a clinician can point out the incongruity between the patient's words and demeanor: "You say you're not depressed, yet you sound so sad," or "It's surprising that you don't sound angry after such an experience." These types of confrontations often produce insights into patients' behavior, conflicts, or feelings without putting the patient on the defensive. Confronting patients with what you observe about their body language does not require conclusions about their motives. Many patients are not able to explain why they feel the way they do. Feedback that asks 'why' tends to place patients on the defensive and requires them to justify their behavior. Confrontations that merely describe what is observed allow patients to think through the conflict or merely shrug their shoulders and go on.

## Doctors Telling Patients the Truth

Patients also have a right to expect truth from doctors. The era in which the doctor could conceal the diagnosis from the patient is long gone. Those who try discover that the patient already knows, often told in the most awkward way by the insurance company, the nurse, or the laboratory technician. Truth telling does not mean telling all that is known, only what the doctor thinks makes a difference to patients plus what patients want to know as reflected by their questions. "I chose to keep my 5 percent probabilities to myself[14]," wrote Hilfiker. Truth telling does not require a confession of every doubt that has ever gone through a human mind. A combination of the reasonable-person standard as viewed by the physician, and the subjective standard based on questions from the patient, usually provides adequate guidelines for what needs to be conveyed.

Telling the truth also does not mean discussing the patient's problem with every friend or family member, even with the patient's permission. In seriously ill patients when multiple family members are involved, the potential for different individuals to interpret the same words differently is enormous. Often it is wise and practical to have the patient or family suggest one person who will keep in touch with you, allowing other family members to convey their questions or concerns through the chosen individual.

How to tell the truth is still an active issue for doctors. Remember that the sixty percent probability of survival is also a forty percent probability of death. A subtle means by which clinicians fail to convey the truth is by the way we express a patient's prognosis. In situations of high risk it is tempting to overestimate the severity of a situation. This approach is sometimes referred to as "hanging crepe." As the term implies, it has been commonly used when dealing with seriously ill patients whose prognosis, despite the best medical care, is poor. Often it is appropriate to give the family a realistic appraisal when the patient has a poor prognosis. However, increasingly this strategy is being used in much less life-threatening situations. Clinicians who use this approach may feel that their partially successful efforts will be viewed as positive, especially if the patient or family is prepared for the worst. Thus clinicians may overemphasize the degree of postoperative pain, the long period of postoperative rehabilitation, the disfiguring character of the surgical scars, or the likelihood of postoperative impotence. This may be done in hopes that patients will be prepared for the worst and delighted at obtaining the usual results. The dangers inherent in this strategy include deterring patients from beneficial procedures, increasing the likelihood of postoperative complications, and undermining the basic doctor-patient relationship.

The desire to provide hope while revealing the essential truth is still an important challenge for the doctor-patient relationship. Helping patients face the truth without losing hope is one of the most difficult and important roles the doctor plays. As Siegel has written and millions have read in his best selling book *Love, Medicine, and Miracles*:

> The word terminal implies a state of mind more than a physical condition, and it turns off the staff's empathy and ability to give the full measure of care needed . . . When physicians run out of remedies, they're likely to give up. They must realize, however, that lack of faith in the patient's ability to heal can severely limit that ability. We should never say 'there's nothing more I can do,' even if it's only to sit down, talk, and help the patient hope and pray[18].

Conveying bad news is usually the most difficult truth to convey. Knowing how much of the truth to tell at one visit is often critical. Patients usually convey by their expressions and questions how much they want to hear now. Truth should often be prescribed in small doses. Physicians must remember, however, to offer the next dose. Alpert and Wittenberg[11] offer a series of recommendations for conveying bad news, including:

Take ample time—nothing is more frustrating and depressing for the patient than a discussion about serious findings without adequate time to ask questions, voice fears, make plans.

Hold the discussion in a private, comfortable place. If the patient desires it, allow close family members to be present.

Have a treatment ready and state it along with the bad news. Ending on a treatment note suggests hope, not hopelessness.

Assure the patient of your continued support and continued presence.

## Doctors Telling Themselves the Truth

Finally, we must recognize that truth telling is commonly thought of as an obligation on the part of the patient to the doctor and the doctor to the patient. However, one of the most important and productive types of truth telling in medicine is our need to be truthful with ourselves. Being truthful with ourselves requires that we acknowledge our own limitations and our own needs. We must set effective limitations on our responsibilities to allow us to satisfy these needs. Setting limits at the career level requires choices about how to utilize our limited time. Clinical care inevitably expands to fill all the time available and then some. The decision to set limits and make decisions about our use of time is critical. As Alpert and Wittenberg have written:

In the beginning the physician often has the energy
needed to grapple with this panorama of demands.
However, if self-expectations are too high, if involvement is too complete, if ability to plan is poor, a weari-
ng out process begins. The symptoms of this process
include a feeling of harassment, an overlay of irri-
tability, a cynical manner, exaggerated hopes of satisfaction from financial gain or material things at times,
depression, and even a resort to drugs or alcohol at
other times[11].

Truth telling also requires that we hold to our
own strongly-held convictions. There is the increasingly frequent situation in clinical medicine in which
the patient's truth and the doctor's truth cannot be
reconciled. Irreconcilable differences may result
when doctors draw the line, refusing to prescribe a
therapy that the patient wants, or when patients refuse to accept medical treatment that the doctor
feels is clearly indicated. Physicians have a right to
refuse to prescribe potentially dangerous therapy, to
say no to requests for additional narcotics, and to
stop testing even when no disease has been identified. Doctors have long learned to live with patients
who ignore their advice. They are now learning to
live with patients who give them more than advice;
they give them orders. When possible, patients
should be presented with options, but doctors must
by necessity be prepared to say no without hostility.
Thus the doctor-patient relationship remains basic
to the practice of medicine. The therapeutic relationship, uncertainty sharing, and truth telling that ideally occur cannot be replaced by modern
technology, no matter how high tech. Ideally, the
doctor-patient relationship serves to complement the
marvels of high-tech medicine. To paraphrase
Naisbitt, what is needed today is both "high tech"
and "high touch[19]." That is a technically competent
clinician who knows how to talk to patients and actually enjoys it.

# REFERENCES

1. Katz J. *The Silent World of Doctor and Patient.* New York: The Free Press, 1984.

2. Brody H. The Lie that Heals: The Ethics of Giving Placebos. Ann of Int Med 1982;97:112–118.

3. Selzer R. *Letters to a Young Doctor.* New York: Simon and Schuster, 1982.

4. Quill TE. Recognizing and adjusting to barriers in doctor-patient communication. *Ann Intern Med* 111:51–57, 1989.

5. Rynearson RR. Touching people (editorial). *J Clin Psychiatry.* 39(6):492, 1978.

6. Balint M. *The Doctor, His Patient and the Illness.* New York: International Universities Press, 1957. P. 1.

7. Cousins N. *Anatomy of an Illness as Perceived by the Patient.* Toronto: Bantam Books, 1981. P. 56–57.

8. Hahn SR, Feiner JS, and Bellin EH. The doctor-patient family relationship. A compensatory alliance. *Ann Intern Med.* 109:884–89, 1988.

9. Groves JE. Taking care of the hateful patient. *N Engl J Med.* 298:883, 1978.

10. Nesheim R. Caring for patients who are not easy to like. *Postgrad Med.* 72(5):255–266, 1982.

11. Alpert JS, Wittenberg SM. *A Clinician's Companion: A Study Guide for Effective and Humane Patient Care.* Boston: Little, Brown, 1986. P. 133–35.

12. Strauss MD (Ed.) *Familiar Medical Quotations*. Boston: Little, Brown, 1968. P. 300.

13. Gutheil TG, Bursztajn H, and Brodsky A. Malpractice prevention through the sharing of uncertainty. *N Engl J Med*. 311:149–51, 1984.

14. Hilfiker D. *Healing the Wounds: A Physician Looks at His Work*. New York: Pantheon Books, 1983.

15. Lipp MR. Respectful Treatment: A Practical Handbook of Patient Care (2nd ed.). New York: Elsevier, 1986.

16. Johnson CG, Levenkron JC, Suchren AL, and Manchester R. Does physician uncertainty affect patient satisfaction. *J Gen Intern Med*. 3:149, 1988.

17. Sokas R. Personal Communication, 1989.

18. Siegel BS. *Love, Medicine and Miracles*. New York: Perennial Library and Row, 1986. P. 38.

19. Naisbitt J. *Megatrends*. New York: Warner Books, 1984. P. 35.

# 14

# *Facing Fallibility*

"If you haven't made any errors that have resulted in death or significant morbidity to one of your patients, you haven't been in practice very long[1]," writes Lipp. Errors are such an intrinsic component of medical practice that the goal of this book is to provide an approach that allows us to analyze why they have occurred and also to respond when they do occur. Throughout we have been discussing errors, and have dealt indepth with errors that we will call errors of implementation. Errors of implementation are those errors we have discussed in the SHADE process of diagnosis, the PESTER process of therapy, and the process of gaining TRUST in the doctor-patient relationship. Errors of implementation are problems that occur in getting the job done—implementing what we intend. To complete our approach to analyzing and categorizing errors, let's turn our attention to other reasons why undesirable results occur. We call these:

Errors of ignorance
Bad outcomes

Errors of ignorance, as opposed to errors of implementation, acknowledge that clinicians must have a great deal of knowledge or facts in order to recognize what needs to be done. Knowledge is a prerequisite to implementation; we need to know before we can use what we know.

Errors of implementation and errors of ignorance are, in theory, preventable. Thus we will call these two types of errors mistakes. In retrospect when we have looked into the reason for an error and concluded that we should have done things differently, a mistake has occurred. Mistakes thus include errors of ignorance and errors of implementation.

Bad outcomes on the other hand may occur even though we have been doing things right—right according to the current medical thinking. Bad outcomes may occur because decision making in medicine is based on probabilities. Even a very high probability of being right implies a small but not zero probability of being wrong. Thus bad outcomes are built into the practice of medicine. They are intrinsic to the way we diagnose and the way we evaluate treatment.

A bad outcome may occur even if the physician was acting "appropriately", practicing according to the current standards. Bad outcomes may occur, for example, when we carefully identify a disease relying on standard laboratory tests that are less than perfect or rule out a disease using testing methods that are less than perfect. Our tests are not usually perfect and neither are our diagnoses. Bad outcomes also may occur when we rely on official recommendations designed to select the best among less than perfect therapies. No therapeutic choice guarantees success, for in medicine there are no guarantees only probabilities. Bad outcomes can be recognized from the answer to the following question asked after you have looked into the reason for an error: "Knowing what you know *now*, should you have done things differently?" If the answer is, "No, I should have done things the same," then a bad outcome, as opposed to a mistake, has occurred.

Having categorized errors as errors of implementation and errors of ignorance, and having distinguished errors from bad outcomes, we are ready to develop a system for categorizing the reasons for undesirable results. Figure 14–1 outlines a flowchart for categorizing the reason for undesirable results. Having recognized an undesirable result you begin by asking, "Knowing what you know now should you have done things differently?" If the answer is no, a bad outcome has occurred. Bad outcomes come in two varieties. Bad outcomes may be the results of medical care or they may be unrelated to medical care. Bad outcomes that are related to medical care will be called adverse medical effects. Bad outcomes, however, may not be related to medical care. Congential abnormalities, death from drug abuse, and sudden cardiac death may occur totally unrelated to medical care. These types of bad outcomes we will call nonmedical effects. Thus the flowsheet asks you to decide, "Did medical care play a role in bringing about the outcome?" If the answer is yes, an adverse medical effect has occurred. If the answer is no, we call the bad outcome a nonmedical effect.

If we decide that a mistake as opposed to a bad outcome has occurred, we need to distinguish two types of mistakes; errors of implementation and errors of ignorance. We have spent most of the book looking at the reason for errors of implementation in the SHADE process of diagnosis, the PESTER process of therapy, and the process of gaining TRUST in the doctor-patient relationship. But what are the sources of errors of ignorance?

## ERRORS OF IGNORANCE

Knowing is not a one time accomplishment, and errors of ignorance are not limited to medical stu-

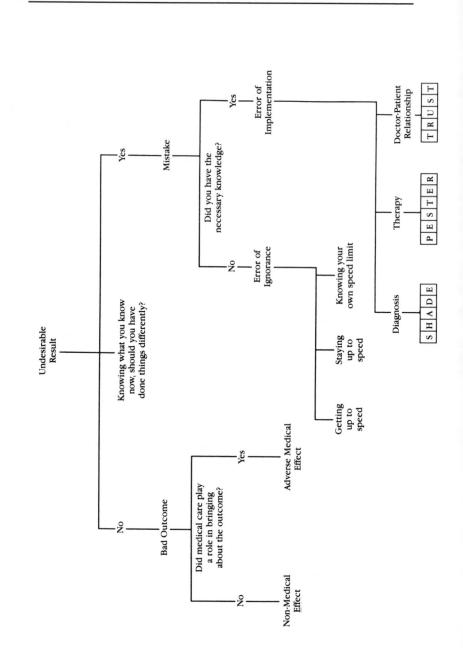

dents. New concepts, new diseases, and new technologies are appearing so fast that many practicing physicians feel more ignorant every year.

There are three basic sources of the errors of ignorance. We will call these failure to:

Get up to speed
Stay up to speed
Know your own speed limit

## Getting Up to Speed

Much of the time spent in medical school, graduate medical education, and continuing medical education is geared toward being sure physicians know the information or facts about diseases, tests, and treatments. For most medical students the most basic fear is not knowing all the facts that "must" be known, not just to pass the boards, but to practice medicine competently.

Knowing what needs to be known is also critical to medical students' sense of control, confidence, and identity as a physician. Thus no one should minimize the need to know the basic facts. However, despite the importance of learning the basic facts, too much emphasis on learning facts is not productive. As Lipp has written, "If you don't know everything, you will kill someone. If you don't know everything, you will be a lousy doctor, and you don't belong in clinical medicine! That, of course, is the Big Lie — and probably the source of more unhappiness and guilt and personal suffering in physicians than all other misbeliefs put together[1]."

Getting up to speed requires hard work but it also requires contemplation. It requires physicians in training to step back, put things they've learned together, and get the big picture. Often there is precious little time in medical school and postgraduate training for such calculated contemplation. Three occasions offer an opportunity for such contemplation—toward the end of the second year and fourth year of medical school and toward the end of residency training. With time to gain perspective at a premium, it is key that students and physicians utilize the time available to prepare for clinical training, residency, and for practice by not simply trying to learn more, but by reviewing, synthesizing, and contemplating what is already known. Facts have a short half life if they are not put into a framework where they can be accessed later. Often reviewing a quality textbook, to read about the common and serious diseases one more time is the best preparation for boards and beyond.

## Staying Up to Speed

Staying up to speed is harder than getting up to speed if we can judge difficulty by success rate. It is all too easy for busy practitioners to deceive themselves into believing that they are practicing quality medicine, especially if most of their patients are appreciative and get better. As Osler wrote, "It is astonishing with how little reading a doctor can practice medicine, but it is not astonishing how badly he can do it[2]."

Whereas most physicians achieve an acceptable standard of knowledge in their chosen field at the end of their postgraduate training, a much smaller percentage remain knowledgeable 15, 30, or 45 years later. Practicing physicians, in fact, probably have more anxiety over their ability to pass tests of knowledge than medical students or residents. Practicing physicians have long resisted compulsory recertification, and only a small percentage show up for voluntary recertification examinations. Paradoxically, students and recent graduates have the most difficulty with errors of implementation due to difficulties using what they know. Experienced physicians, on the other hand, often make errors of ignorance, failing to be aware of entire fields of new knowledge, new techniques to answer critical diagnostic questions, or new available effective therapies.

There's no easy answer for keeping up to speed except time and attention. A few tips, however, may make the job a little more efficient and pleasurable. First, think about your own learning style—do you learn best from lectures, reading, looking at videotapes on your own television, active group discussions, or other ways. A mixture of these may make sense to sustain or enliven the process, but for day-to-day keeping up, you need a process that fits into your lifestyle and learning style. Catching grand rounds before seeing patients in the hospital, listening to tapes on the way home, or reading journals with your feet up before bed may each fit some lifestyles better than others. There are so many ways of keeping up to speed today that physicians should be able to develop an approach that fits their learning style and lifestyle.

Equally important to consider are your goals for continuing medical education and to be sure that they are consistent with your philosophy and type of practice. If you intend to specialize in a rapidly changing field, concentrating on applying the latest in medical technology, then reading the latest research journals may be critically important. However, such a goal requires awareness of the limitations of clinical research. At least wait until you've seen the letters to the editor before putting it into practice. If your goal is to practice competently in a broader field, your aim for continuing medical education may be to know the consensus and the official recommendations. Often clinical reviews in major medical journals and periodic updates, such as the American College of Physicians' Medical

Knowledge Self Assessment Program (MKSAP), will
bring you up to speed while maintaining enough
caution to avoid propelling you beyond the consensus. Often putting aside time every few years to repeat a process like MKSAP will allow you to gain
not only the facts but the perspective on how medicine is changing over the years.

## Knowing Your Own Speed Limit

Knowing your own speed limit, your limits of information, concepts, and skills is critical to practicing
medicine. As Lipp has written, "The only truly terri-
ble things that happens in association with limitations comes as a consequence of refusing to
recognize their existence and substituting arrogance for humility[1]." Arrogance abounds in medicine and can only be tolerated when matched by an
equal degree of competence. Perhaps there is no
more dangerous combination than arrogance and ignorance. Knowing your speed limit means knowing
when to ask for help, when to look it up, and when
to limit the type of problems you take on. Knowing
what you can do and what you can't is an essential
feature of quality care. Doctors readily admit that
they are not expert in all diseases. They less readily
acknowledge that they are unable to treat all patients, especially those whose disease falls within
their area of expertise. Inability to acknowledge
failure, seek second opinions, and openly discuss
frustrations is a sure formula for disaster. Respected colleagues often have the distance and ob-
jectivity to readily identify the psychological
barriers that close contact obscures. Those who fail
to recognize when they can't help are doomed to
further failure.
Errors of ignorance are not limited to medical
students. They recur in new ways throughout a med-

ical career. Getting up to speed, staying up to speed, and knowing your own speed limit are critical to getting where you're going.

## WHEN MISTAKES OCCUR

Mistakes, whether they be errors of ignorance or errors of implementation, are an everyday part of clinical practice. As Hilfiker writes, "As a student I was simply not aware that the sort of mistakes I would eventually make in practice actually happen to competent physicians. As far as I can remember from my student's experience on the hospital wards, the only doctors who ever made mistakes were the much maligned, 'LMDs' local medical doctors[3]."

Mistakes are an inherent part of medical practice. Thus it is essential to have an approach to dealing with errors. Faced with the occurrence of an error what should the physician do? Before exploring some positive approaches to this question, let us first look at how physicians often try, counterproductively, to deal with their own mistakes. Mizrahi, who has studied the ways housestaff at a "middle of the road" university training program handled their errors, found that these physicians often used three potentially destructive mechanisms[4]:

Denial
Discounting
Distancing

When these house staff were asked about errors they and their colleagues had made, they readily acknowledged the occurrence of errors. Over half acknowledged serious and even fatal errors during the first two months of internship. These errors included putting patients into congestive heart failure, rupturing organs, causing renal failure, and sending patients with acute coronary artery disease home. Despite the fact that these residents appear to recognize errors, they tended to deny that the error could have been prevented, thereby classifying most of their undesirable results as bad outcomes rather than errors or mistakes. Bad outcomes are the most comfortable category, because as one resident said, "It is just the nature of the business[4]." Some residents practiced a severe form of denial called repression; they couldn't remember the occurrence of the error. Denial is counterproductive if it keeps us from analyzing the sources of errors and learning from their occurrence.

Discounting, or transfer of responsibility, for preventing a mistake was also a common means of dealing with mistakes. Errors were blamed on the system, "You have to take care of so much 'garbage' in this place you don't have time to check on every little thing and a lot of times things are missed," said one resident. Blaming superiors was also a common means of denial of responsibility. One resident described a patient who had "questionable" cardiac arrest who was transferred to the cardiology service, saying,

> I went up and asked them (superiors in Cardiology) if I could put a monitor on him and they said not unless the resident thought it was needed. It kind of got lost in the wash. The resident didn't spend a lot of time on him and he agreed not to put one on him and then the patient had chest pains and in the morning he died[4].

In another form of discounting, patients too may be blamed. They may be regarded as poor historians despite the physician's lack of effort or skills in securing the history. They may be called uncooperative or noncompliant when the physician's instructions were not clear or his or her prescription produced side effects. Even worse, patients may be labelled as "goamers," "crocks," "turkeys," or other pejorative terms as a prelude to placing all responsibility for mistakes on the patients themselves. Carmichael describes another form of blaming the patient characterized by much bravado. "How dare the patient have a serious complication when I have done such a wonderful operation made a spectacular diagnosis, etc[5]!"

A third means of dealing with mistakes has been labelled distancing. In this form of defense mechanism the physician justifies the mistake as actually a bad outcome by saying, "Everyone makes mistakes." "It couldn't be helped." The opposite of distancing also occurs. In hindsight many bad outcomes that could not be prevented are seen as mistakes. In fact, the "retrospectoscope" may be the most powerful diagnostic tool in medicine. Hindsight bias has repeatedly been shown to influence the way other people view our errors, and even how we ourselves view them. "Why didn't I see that . . . why didn't I ask that," may seem obvious questions only after the fact. It is important to avoid both the extremes of instantly blaming ourselves and instantly distancing ourselves from blame.

All of these reasons and ways of dealing with error may be valid at times, but they often leave physicians unable to learn from mistakes and at times unable to deal with them. Hilfiker writes, "Unable to admit our mistakes, we physicians are cut off from healing. We cannot ask for forgiveness, and we get none. We are thwarted, stunted; we do not grow[3]."

How else can physicians deal with errors other than denial, discounting, and distancing. There are three steps necessary for dealing with an error:

Recognizing: Acknowledging the error
Rectifying: Making right what can be restored

Resolving: Forgiving what can be forgiven and resolving not to repeat the error.

At first glance none of these are currently possible in medicine. Malpractice lawyers stress denial
and physicians routinely practice denial. We rarely
hear of acknowledging errors and assuming responsibility. Making right what can be restored in medicine may not be possible, except financially once
the damage is done. Resolving is impossible and forgiveness cannot occur if no error has ever been acknowledged. However, if we look again there are a
number of ways we can deal effectively with errors.
First, we can accept responsibility as a way to acknowledge the error. As Alpert writes, "... if the vic-
tories are the physician's, so are the defeats[6]."
Acceptance of responsibility acknowledges that the
physician must deal with the problem. Acknowledging blame at least at this stage, is not usually appropriate. Rather, acknowledging responsibility, that an
error has been made and will be dealt with is more
important.

Attempts to rectify must focus on the potential
consequences of the error as rapidly as possible in
an attempt to minimize the consequences. Errors of
ignorance, errors of implementation, and adverse
medical effects all share some things in common—
Physicians have a role in their occurrence and have
a responsibility to recognize them early. Not all errors or adverse effects lead to disaster; some are
near misses that are caught just in time; others are
wrong decisions whose impact is minimized by
catching them early and dealing with them
promptly.

Regardless of the success of these efforts, to
recognize and rectify the errors and adverse effects,
we must analyze the reasons for the error and determine why it occurred. We have discussed a diagnostic approach to analyzing and categorizing

undesirable results that helps us determine why it happened. Distinguishing the type of error is key since there is a different therapy for each diagnosis. Errors of ignorance due to lack of knowledge require more education. Mistakes taken seriously are often the best teachers. If the diagnosis is an error of implementation this book provides a means to pinpoint the problem(s) and offer suggestions for improvement. Analyzing the 'whys' will hopefully prevent a reoccurrence. If the diagnosis is an adverse medical effect then we can rightfully feel free of guilt without having to rely on denial, discounting, or distancing.

Having recognized and acknowledged the error; having sought to rectify the problem and minimize its impact; and having analyzed and learned from the error, we can hope to resolve the problem in our own minds. Having dealt with our own errors we can expect compassion from others and a freedom from guilt.

We in medicine can do better. We can aim to minimize the medical mistakes that are due to errors of ignorance and errors of implementation. We can aim to accept the adverse effect that is part of the practice of medicine. By definition we will not be perfect. In the end, the goal is to be able to look the patient or the family in the eye and honestly say, "I did the best I could."

## REFERENCES

1. Lipp MR. Respectful Treatment: A Practical Handbook of Patient Care (2nd ed.). New York: Elsevier, 1986.

2. Osler, Sir William. *Aphorisms From His Bedside Teachings and Writings*. In WB Bean, (Ed.). New York: Henry Schuman, 1950. P. 36.

3. Hilfiker D. *Healing the Wounds: A Physician Looks at His Work.* New York: Pantheon Books, 1985. P. 83.

4. Mizrahi T. Managing medical mistakes: Ideology insularity and accountability among internists in-training. *Soc Sci Med* 19(2):135–146, 1984.

5. Carmichael DH. Learning medical fallibility. *South Med J.* 78(2):1–3, 1985.

6. Alpert JS, Wittenberg SM. *A Clinician's Companion: A Study Guide for Effective and Humane Patient Care.* Boston: Little, Brown, 1986. P. 30.

# Appendix

In order to put together the approach to identifying the source of errors presented in *Minimizing Medical Mistakes*, see Figure 14–1. The flowchart is designed to help separate bad outcomes from errors, and errors of ignorance from errors of implementation. Once an error is categorized as an error of implementation we can further categorize the errors using the type of problems identified in the SHADE process of diagnosis, the PESTER process of therapy, and the process of gaining TRUST through the doctor-patient relationship.

The appendix contains a checklist of the errors of implementation that we have identified.

## SHADE—THE DIAGNOSTIC PROCESS

**S**ymptoms: Chief complaint
**H**unch: Hypothesis
**A**lternatives: Differential diagnosis
**D**isease Identification: Hypothesis testing
**E**xplanation: Explanation of disease and clinical manifestations

## Step 1: Symptoms

*Rule of Thumb*
> Anchor: Focusing on a chief complaint

*Problem Using*
> Premature closure: Failing to obtain the big picture

*Potential Mistakes*

> Failure to recognize the patient's true purpose for
> seeking medical care
> Failure to clarify confusion
> Failure to maximize and evaluate reliability
> Failure to obtain the data accessible through nonver-
> bal communication such as body language
> Failure to re-examine the original focus

## Step 2: Hunch

*Rule of Thumb*
> Representativeness: Think of a disease pattern
> that matches the patient's symptom pattern

*Problem Using*
> Lack of experience using disease patterns

*Potential Mistakes*

> Failure to recognize incomplete or modified pat-
> terns due to early presentation, multiple diseases,
> or partial treatment
> Failure to circumvent barriers to pattern recogni-
> tion due to what we expect to see, don't wish to
> see, or are too familiar to see
> Failure to obtain the missing piece(s) of the pattern
> due to a patient's denial

## Step 3: Alternatives

*Rule of Thumb*
>    Availability: Develop a limited list of alternatives
>    that comes to mind because of their association
>    through pathophysiology or through clinical
>    associations.

*Problem Using*
>    Failure to make a systemic search of memory utiliz-
>    ing disease categories and clinical checklists to
>    making alternatives more available.

*Potential Mistakes*

>    Failure to consider diseases known to present with
>    misleading manifestations due to medical
>    mirages, or masquerades
>    Failure to consider common diseases presenting
>    with unusual features
>    Looking for rare diseases or zebras without a good
>    reason.

## Step 4: Disease Identification

*Rule of Thumb*
>    Hypothesis Testing: Use positive test to rule in a
>    disease and negative tests to rule out a disease.

*Problem Using*
>    Failure to maximize the value of the physical exam-
>    ination as a collection of diagnostic tests.

*Potential Mistakes*

>    Ordering tests without asking "Why is the test being
>    ordered?"

Failure to estimate the pretest probability of a disease before ordering a test.
Failure to fully utilize negative test results.
Failure to recognize the limitations of positive and negative test results defined by a range of normal.
Over-reliance on the weight of the evidence and the susceptibility to information overload when combining test results.
Ordering tests because we can't stand to wait, have a need to be complete, are scared by lawsuit, or fail to recognize when enough is enough.
Failure to understand, what a disease is?

## Step 5: Explanation

### *Rule of Thumb*
Principle of Parsimony: Tie together the clinical manifestations, disease, and the cause with one explanation.

### *Problem Using*
Failure to listen to the patient for help linking together the clinical manifestations, disease, and the cause(s).

### *Potential Mistakes*
Failure to systematically determine whether a disease is actually the explanation of the patient's symptoms.
Failure to consider multiple diseases in the same individual and recognize that not all diseases produce clinical manifestations.
Failure to acknowledge the uncertainty that remains.

# PESTER: THE THERAPEUTIC PROCESS

Prediction
Effectiveness
Safety
Therapeutic Decisions
Execution
Reflection

## Prediction

Analyzing the risk of developing disease and the prognosis once disease develops:

Failure to provide prevention
Failure to recognize how lead time bias and length bias may produce an apparent success of early intervention
Failure to recognize that relative risk does not indicate the magnitude of the risk and that risk factors may interact to multiply the risk
Failure to accurately assess the severity of disease as part of prognosis
Failure to accurately assess the urgency of treatment as part of prognosis

## Effectiveness

Evaluating the efficacy, effectiveness, and cost-effectiveness of potential therapies

Failure to recognize the inherent limitation of controlled clinical trials, including nonrandom selection of patients and difficulty assessing long-term and secondary effects
Failure to recognize the limitation of clinical experience due to patient selection, selective follow-up, and biased recall of results

Failure to understand the meaning of the concepts
of cost effectiveness—including cost savings,
cost effective, and most cost effective

Failure to appreciate how cost effectiveness in clinical practice may be influenced by how a technology is utilized

**Safety:**

Assess the safety of potential therapies for the individual patient.

Failure to assess the probability of side effects taking into account the treatment's mechanism of action, margin of safety, plus the patient's propensity
for side effects and drug interactions due to multiple drug use

Failure to assess the severity of side effects taking
into account the potential for morbidity and mortality, the ease of detection or reversibility, and
the timing of occurrence

Failure to recognize the existence of unpredictable
risks of treatment from new therapies and for established therapies used for new indications

**Therapeutic Decisions:**

Developing and communicating physician
recommendations and engaging patients in informed
consent.

Failure to view physician recommendations and
informed consent as two separate and required
parts of therapeutic decision-making

Failure to recognize problems in developing
subjective probabilities, including overreliance on
imaginability and the gambler's fallacy that
chance runs in streaks

Failure to recognize how patients' utilities may differ from physicians' utilities for potential outcomes, including distortions produced by the dread effect; the utilities patients place on time; and the value of quality of life

Failure to recognize when physicians or patients strongly deviate from risk neutrality, including the influence of the insurance effect leading to risk aversion and the longshot effect leading to risk seeking

Failure to recognize that decision making may be influenced by how data is conveyed, including use of the dread effect and the framing effect

Failure to recognize impaired capacity to decide and dealing with impaired judgment

## Execution of Therapy:

Implementing what the physician intends and the patient desires.

Failure to recognize common physician's misconceptions, including difficulty in predicting compliance, overstressing education in pathophysiology, and failing to clarify and simplify the treatment

Failure to recognize common patient behaviors, including the complications of common sense; the fallacy of following orders; the legacy of leftovers; the sequelae of spectacular results; allowing annoyance to prevent adherence; and failing to follow-up when the problem extends beyond the patient

Failure to stress changes in behavior based on principles of behavior modification

## Reflection:

Assessing the results of therapy in light of the patient's response.

Failure to determine whether the treatment was actually executed

Failure to rethink the diagnosis to determine whether the disease and the cause were correct

Failure to ask whether the therapy is getting to the patient. Is the patient taking the therapy properly and is the therapy bioavailable?

Failure to ask whether the treatment is getting to the site of action. Is the therapy being maintained at therapeutic levels and is the therapy penetrating to the site of action?

Failure to ask whether the treatment is having its intended biological effect. Is the treatment producing effects that counter its intended effect, and is tolerance to the therapy developing?

Failure to ask whether the treatment is having its intended therapeutic effect. Are there acceptable alternatives or should we settle for a partial response?

## TRUST: THE DOCTOR-PATIENT RELATIONSHIP

### Therapeutic Relationships:

Utilizing the doctor-patient relationship to achieve the placebo effect without the placebo.

Failure to recognize patients who do not seek a therapeutic relationship

Failure to recognize patients who seek to utilize the doctor-patient relationship to fulfill other agendas

Failure to recognize and be prepared to deal with types of patients that doctors find difficult

Failure to recognize situations where the doctor-patient relationship hinders the recognition of new problems

## Uncertainty Sharing:

Utilizing the doctor-patient relationship to share the inevitable uncertainty of medical care.

Use of excessive testing in a fruitless effort to remove uncertainty
Superimposing certainty as a means of dealing with uncertainty
Failure to anticipate system failure and provide a safety net
Failure to use uncertainty sharing as a basis for a therapeutic alliance

## Truth:

Utilizing the doctor-patient relationship to allow the patient and the doctor to recognize and communicate truth.

Failure to help patients tell doctors the truth by acknowledging their true feelings and true motives
Failure to tell patients the truth by communicating the essential diagnostic and therapeutic situation while maintaining hope
Failure of physicians to tell themselves the truth by failing to recognize and plan for their own needs and failing to say no to unreasonable patient expectations without hostility

# *Index*

# Index